contained within this document, including, but not limited to, —
errors, omissions, or inaccuracies.

Table of Contents

Chapter 16 Making Things Pleasurable and Fun!

Conclusion

Description

Learning how to master self-discipline truly is the art of learning how to win at life. By listening to this entire audiobook, you have filled your life with all of the knowledge required to tap into the tools that the most successful men on earth are using in their own lives. Knowing how to have such a high sense of self-awareness that you can discipline yourself to live life in a specific way that has you operating at peak performance at all times takes a special level of skill and mastery that not everyone is willing to tap into. Of course, everyone has access to this information and the ability to develop these skills, yet most people are too lazy and unwilling to truly make the difference in their own lives.

If you apply even just half of these skills in your life, you are going to be ahead of so many people who are constantly sitting around making excuses and unwilling to genuinely make a change in their lives. This means that even just applying half of this knowledge is going to set you so much further ahead than a vast majority of the population. If you take this all the way and truly embody self-discipline mastery by applying all of these tips and steps into your life, you have the capacity to put yourself into that 1% of the population who performs better than anybody else. This means more money, more freedom, more success, and more personal achievement.

If you find that you really have a hard time committing to these new practices, get yourself a friend who is also mastering self-discipline and start holding each other accountable. For many people, just having someone else who can relate is the best way for them to stay committed and keep growing because they know that they are not alone. Remember, you are the sum of the three to five people that you hang out with, so if you really want to keep these changes going, hang out with better people. Find yourself people who are genuinely interested in bettering themselves, befriend them, and keep your social circle healthy and strategic. Your future self will thank you.

This guide will focus on the following:

- Self-confident mind
- Pros and cons of self-discipline
- Why constraints are necessary
- How to build self-discipline
- Self-discipline strategies
- Military discipline and self-discipline
- Your friendship with pain
- Pareto principle
- Look for micro improvements
- The psychology of self-discipline
- Self-confidence boost
- The triad of success

- Making things pleasurable and fun!... AND MORE!!!

Introduction

Self-discipline is exactly what it says—the ability to discipline oneself. It is the ability to know what to do in situations and the fortitude to actually do what is correct in the situation. It is a habit that is vital to daily success. Truly successful people are usually highly disciplined people.

No one is born with the ability to truly self-discipline. Babies only care about being taken care of and having their needs met. As children grow, their parents are in charge of their discipline— at least in the beginning. Parents make the rules, and children follow them because small children lack the thought processes needed to make good decisions on a regular basis. Small children only see the here-and-now, the immediate gratification. They do not know and do not care that a bigger, better reward might be in store for them if they wait patiently. They lack foresight. As children grow up, they begin to see the reasoning behind their parent's rules. They begin to make choices that mirror the choices their parents have made for them in the past. They show that they are learning to discipline themselves. At this point, the parents may begin to step back a little and to loosen the reins. They may allow the child a bit more freedom in making decisions, with the understanding that the parent is available if the choice turns out to be unfavorable. In this way, the child learns in the safety of the home and with the protection of the parents to make good choices and formulate good decisions. The child learns to self-discipline.

In a perfect world, this is the way children would be raised. Unfortunately, this is the real world and not a perfect one. The problem is not that parents do not care about their children—it is that many parents do not know how to teach the art of self-discipline to their children. Maybe the parents are not self-disciplined, maybe the parents feel the child will learn it eventually, or maybe the parents simply do not want to let go complete control over the child. For whatever reason, most children are not taught self-discipline as a way of life and reach adulthood with no clue of how to be in charge of themselves.

However, the good news is that self-discipline can be learned. While best learned while growing up, as a part of learning to be an adult, it is possible to learn as an adult and begin to practice self-discipline skills immediately. Moreover, by learning self-discipline in adulthood, the person has a total buy-in to the idea. This is a personal choice. This is something that needs to be done in order to enjoy a better life. This does not mean that learning self-discipline as an adult will be easier or faster, but at least, the adult who makes the conscious choice to become more self-disciplined has a personal stake in its success.

Self-discipline is nothing more than managing one's own personal affairs. It is a way of behaving where people automatically choose to do what should be done, as opposed to what would more preferably be done. It is studying for a test instead of going to a party. It is washing dirty laundry on a regular basis, so that clean clothes are always available. It is following a budget so that future financial goals can be realized. Self-discipline is that inner voice controlling outward actions. It is using willpower to become mentally tough enough to control one's actions by oneself.

Almost anything that a person does to focus on an end goal rather than immediate satisfaction is self-discipline. The underlying problem is that it is always much easier to follow the path of impulse. Impulse is fun. Impulse is now. Impulse allows for joining the group and having a fun night on the town instead of studying and doing laundry. Impulse is the exact opposite of self-discipline.

Granted impulse is much more fun than discipline. Impulse gives the opportunity to have fun and be with friends. Impulse means staying up late and sleeping in tomorrow. Impulse means spending the extra money on the desirable frivolous toy and not saving anything this week. But impulse will not finish homework, wash clothes, follow a schedule, or save money. Self-discipline is needed for those things. Does this mean that impulse has no place in a life ruled by self-discipline? Absolutely not! Impulsive action is an almost automatic action. A cake is meant to be eaten. Self-discipline should never be so rigid that people go through life acting like little robots with no feelings and no desires. Everyone wants a cake. Having self-discipline just means eating one slice of cake and not the whole cake.

Practicing self-discipline requires great self-knowledge. Think about that for a minute. How can anything be changed if all the facts are not known? Imagine walking into a kitchen and seeing a small child and a puddle of water. The first instinct would be to believe the child spilled something. But what if someone else spilled something and then left the puddle on the floor? What if the pipe under the sink is leaking? Without knowing all the facts, there is no way to come to the correct conclusion. The path to self-discipline begins with knowing, and admitting the existence of, personal weaknesses. Everyone has those things they would rather not do. People would rather not admit to being imperfect, but all are and must be prepared to admit to imperfections to be able to begin the journey to self-discipline. The next step is to be prepared to move everyday temptations out of the way. This is usually easier said than done, but it must be done to begin along the path toward self-discipline properly. Once ready to begin, make sure to set clear, realistic goal and make a plan to achieve them. Do not be afraid to set several smaller goals as opposed to one large ultimate goal. Nothing worthwhile is ever reached in one straight path. There will be roadblocks and pitfalls along the way that will necessitate reworking the plan. So, it may be better to start with smaller goals that will give a sense of accomplishment that will help ease traveling this path.

Keep the plan simple. Self-discipline does not need to be complicated. The idea of self-discipline itself is actually a very simple concept. The plan to get to self-discipline should not be overly complicated. The plan to reach self-discipline should be as simple as possible while encompassing all aspects needed to reach the goal. A complicated plan may be impossible to achieve and will probably lead to defeat—and giving up is not an option on the road to self-discipline.

Self-discipline is a powerful tool to possess. Self-discipline is a positive force in life. It does not mean giving up those things that make life satisfying; but rather using innate strength and creativity to achieve desired goals. With self-discipline, life is more enjoyable, and the little cheats that help make life enjoyable when people have the self-discipline to learn to enjoy these little cheats only occasionally. Again, it is not necessary to completely give up cake; just do not eat the whole thing!

Self-disciplined people do not deprive themselves, but they use focus to stay on track when goals conflict with one another. Let us imagine that friends want to have fun tonight with a pub crawl. Let us also imagine there is a huge chemistry test tomorrow. The self-disciplined person would stay home and study chemistry, thus giving better odds to getting a good grade and not worrying about the risk of oversleeping and missing the test altogether. The bars will still be there another time.

People who have a high level of self-discipline are more satisfied with themselves and how their life is going. Self-discipline allows for a better sense of self and a higher level of self-esteem. Life is not out of control. Life has meaning beyond today. Worthwhile goals are in sight in the future—and this works in a cycle. Creating goals and making a plan to achieve them leads to a higher sense of self-control. A higher sense of self-control leads to more goal setting and plan making. The cycle just keeps going around.

Self-discipline allows for more time being able to do the things that will bring satisfaction and less of the things that provide no growth or satisfaction. Self-disciplined people set a goal and work toward it. Self-disciplined people are proactive, not reactive. This means they anticipate problems and work to prevent them, rather than trying to solve a problem when it occurs. Proactive people spend time every day wondering 'what if?'. What if the car does not start tomorrow? What if the washing machine breaks down? What if the tree in the backyard falls into the house? Proactive people imagine scenarios and decide on a plan of action before it is needed. If the plan is never needed, then at least there is a plan in place. Reactive people, on the other hand, spend a lot of time doing things that are not producing a future goal. Reactive people react when the problem occurs. They have no preset plan in place. If the car does not start one morning, then they scramble to find an alternate means of transportation for the day. The proactive person might give up eating lunch out every day in favor of brown-bagging lunch then saving that money for a down payment on a house. That is self-discipline. The reactive person will suddenly start scrambling trying to dig up down payment money for a house when the monthly rent increases yet again.

While missing restaurant lunches in order to save money for that future house might seem negative at the moment, it is positive in the long run. With a bit of sacrificing a future goal is achieved. Focusing on daily choices makes living more in the moment than looking toward the future. So, while planning a daily brown-bag lunch might seem like an in-the-moment choice, it is really a part of a long-term goal. Deciding on a different restaurant each day is truly in the moment—and when the goal is achieved, a tremendous sense of satisfaction replaces any feelings of deprivation that may have been lingering.

Boundaries are not scary things, but rather necessary limits to achieving a future goal. Boundaries are needed to achieve the level of self-control needed to become fully self-disciplined. Setting boundaries require knowing exactly what the future goals are and how to follow a path to achieve them. This allows the self-disciplined person to understand themselves better than most people, to be much more comfortable in their own skin than most people. This also allows the self-disciplined person to know exactly what lengths they are capable of achieving in order to reach a goal.

Moreover, becoming self-disciplined will showcase who is a friend and who is not. True friends will assist in achieving goals. True friends will not try to block the hard work needed to become self-disciplined. By making the conscious decision to become self-disciplined, the sad truth of reality means that not everyone can stay around. But the self-disciplined person has the power to create the world as they want it to be.

Self-discipline takes an extreme amount of energy to achieve. It is not just choosing to be self-disciplined—it must be constantly worked at, and that takes energy. This will require good lifestyle practices. Eat healthily, sleep regularly, exercise when possible— all these activities will energize the body and mind and make working toward the goal of self-discipline more easily attainable.

Chapter 1 Self-confident Mind

In a purely scientific sense, hypnosis is related to different states of consciousness or awareness. We have a waking state or a state in which we are fully awake, alert and alive to real-world experiences. There is an awareness of what we experience in and around us. We move from different states of consciousness all through the day. For instance, you are enjoying a relaxing aroma massage treatment, and you begin to feel drowsy, your mind is roaming or subtly shifting from one state of consciousness into another.

Simply put, hypnosis is an altered state of awareness or being, which we move in and out of throughout the day. It occurs even when our eyes are wide open and can be induced without the use of words. For instance, you can be hypnotized simply by staring at a subject continuously. The most important aspect of hypnosis – it diminishes a person's ability to think rationally, evaluate information critically and make independent decisions.

Covert hypnosis is when an attempt is made to communicate with the subject's unconscious mind without the subject knowing that he or she will be put through hypnosis. It comprises a string of technique such as conversational hypnosis or NLP (neuro-linguistic programming), body language and other powerful communication and interaction strategies.

The primary objective of covert hypnosis is to gradually change an individual's behavior at a subconscious level to lead the subject into believing that they changed their mind on their own accord. You simply lead them into believing that they weren't influencer or manipulated by changed their mind on their own.

When covert hypnosis is successfully performed, the subject isn't aware that he or she is being hypnotized. There is considerable debate about the fine line between conventional hypnotism and covert hypnotism. While standard hypnotism is about drawing the focus of the subject, covert hypnotism is primarily about relaxing the subject a bit or softening their stand by using deception, confusion, interruption and a series of other techniques.

Proven Covert Hypnosis Techniques

Here are some forms of covert hypnosis techniques for beginners

1. Deception

Deception is one of the most commonly practiced covert hypnosis techniques to lead the subject into doing what you want without them knowing about your real intentions. For instance, you may want a close friend to give up the addiction and resort to plain deception to lead them away from their addiction triggers or suggest something false without making them catch your true intentions of making them give up alcohol or drugs.

As a practiced hypnotist, you create an illusion or sense of false reality to help the subject believe something you want them to. We have all been susceptible to deception at some point or the other. There is a tendency of believing fictional information without ever asking for details.

Clairvoyants, psychics, and hypnotists used this method generously to create an illusion by gaining the explicit trust of the subject through clever rapport-building techniques.

2. Eye Contact Clues

People almost always display a particular body language type that reflects their deepest thoughts and feelings. Hackneyed as it sounds, "Eyes are truly windows to one's soul." Analyzing an individual's body language (especially their eyes) will award you with a good sense of how a particular word, action, sound, image or emotion is perceived by him or her.

The subject is read based on the direction's his or her eyes are darting in. Examine the subject's eyes thoroughly for cues. This technique is more complicated than it sounds and needs plenty of practice.

3. Misdirection

This covert hypnosis technique is widely used by magicians all over the world to manipulate their audience or create an illusion.

Magicians sneakily use the power of misdirection to distract their audience's attention to another point of focus to perform a quick action that they wish to hide.

For instance, if you are attempting to get the subject to do something by directly sowing the suggestion, they are more consciously aware of your intentions. However, if you are accomplishing the same goal, you distract their attention elsewhere and make the same suggestion worded in another context.

4. Submodalities

There is great variance between the responses of different to the same information. This can be detected by the manipulator using several submodalities (under various contexts) to generate the desired response. Look for voice tone, body language, facial expressions and eyes cues. When the use of certain words or actions creates positive submodalities, you can continue using them to invoke specific feelings or emotions.

5. Generalized Reading

Generalized or warm reading is a covert hypnosis technique based on making generalized observations or statements that could be applicable for just about anyone that do not take into account unique observations or responses gained from the subject.

Fortune tellers, psychic and clairvoyants use a lot of this technique to manipulate their clients into believing that the readings are unique to them, when in fact, these are general observations that can be applicable for just about any person.

For instance, "You are an ambitious person who also strives for happiness, contentment and inner peace. You've learned and evolved from your past experiences. You have overcome your past mistakes to look forward to new and exciting life ahead." You can ask any person to read this, and he or she will end up believing this was written only with him or her in mind. It leads the subject's mind to believe that it is about him or her since they are unique.

Warm readings can be used as icebreakers to establish a rapport of trust with the subject (by making seemingly accurate statements) before they begin to talk. This gives you the advantage to build upon the all too accurate beginning statement.

6. Hot Reading

Hot reading differs from general or warm readings in a manner that you have some prior information about the subject (which he or she is completely unaware of), which completely amazes them.

You've got to find a way to obtain important bits of information about a person without him or knowing about it, which can be tricky. The subject will then be led into believing that you have been blessed with supernatural or psychic abilities.

7. Cold Observations

While warm observations involve making generalized statements that can be applicable to everyone and hot observations are sneakily obtaining specific information about a person to use it to your advantage, cold observations are made based on your initial impression about a person by closely studying them. You then build upon the general statements by making more specific statements based on their responses.

It is regularly used by mentalists, psychics, and spiritualists to form an illusion that can accurately read a person's mind or perform telepathy. Subjects are led into believing that they are indeed everything they are told they are by the manipulator.

It comprises making vague statements after making a few first impression observations of an individual, which can easily be acquired after practicing a few people reading and analyzing skills. For example, you can simply say to your subject, "I have a feeling you are a self-assured and confident individual although you tend to hesitate at times based on past experiences." You wait for a response from the subject.

The subject can come up with a bunch of responses such as, "yes, you're right. I am generally confident and expressive but tend to be held back by past experiences" (which means they are generally confident people), "Oh yes, I do tend to reflect a lot on my past actions" (which means they are more shy and hesitant than self-assured and confident). Once they respond to a general statement, you can use their response to make more specific or direct statements about the person.

Ericksonian Hypnosis Theory

This technique comprises using stories, examples and anecdotes for eliminating the wall of resistance built by our subconscious mind. The hypnotizer or manipulator narrates a story, which ends with a moral that the manipulator desires to convey.

The subject's subconscious mind builds a connection or deep relationship with different aspects of the story. You lead the subject into emotionally linking with the story that sounds similar to the situation they are in currently.

This is s strategy for making indirect suggestions using a story to distract or divert the conscious mind, thus leaving the unconscious more receptive to suggestions.

Power-Packed Conversational Hypnosis Techniques

One form of covert hypnosis that can be used to manipulate someone into what you want is conversational hypnosis. It helps you establish an immediate connection with the other person so you can almost mind read them and lead them to do as you desire.

Among other things, conversational hypnosis gives you the ability to alter a person's state of consciousness right there and then, while driving them into a hypnotic trance. It will get people to obey what you are telling them to do without giving it a logical thought. Conversational hypnosis can be used as a tool for changing a person's behavior and getting them to act on your command. Here are a few time-tested secrets of conversational hypnosis unlocked.

1. Sharpen Your State of Awareness Recognition

To be an ace hypnotizer, you need to be fully aware of or identify trance signals in others. This becomes even more complex when the signals are subtle. Practice enhancing your state of consciousness or awareness so you can better recognize signals of other people changing states of awareness.

Once you gain expertise in the art of being aware of your state of consciousness, it will be easier to gain awareness of the slightest detail around you. Your senses will be open and receptive for quickly catching on to any changes you spot in the immediate environment.

2. Build on It

In this technique of conversational hypnosis, what you are actually doing is slowly sowing a seed of thought or idea in the mind of the other person, which you intend to keep growing over a period of time, one bit at a time.

It starts by asking the person to change something really tiny. Then build on that chain by requesting more and more change. Start with something simple and non-complicated during each session of hypnosis. To make them reach a gradual state of intense trace, gradually and progressively build upon the simple or easy request.

3. Controlling with the Voice

You have to have a distinct tone of voice for trance and nontrance states if you really wish to have a powerful effect on the mind of a person. During the entire hypnosis process, you must progressively move into your special trance tonality.

The idea is to clearly distinguish between your voices when the person transcends through different states of consciousness. Thus, the voice can be slightly lighter in a less intense state of trance and deeper when the trance state is more intense. This way you can control the movement of your subject from one state of consciousness to another simply by using your voice at will. They can be led to move from one state of awareness into another through the power of your voice alone.

4. Repetition

This is a form of controlling the mind through repeated exposure to a thought, idea or behavior pattern. Repetition is a covert hypnotic manipulation tactic used to expose your subject to the same idea or notion again and again until it is deeply embedded into their subconscious mind, and they start believing the notion of being true.

5. Compounding Effect

This technique simply means that each time your idea receives a positive response from the subject; you follow it up with a more powerful one. You are basically building on your last success point. When a suggestion works, you prim up the next one and have it ready for acceptance (greater odds of it being accepted if the earlier suggestion has been received positively).

In the event that your suggestion is met with a negative response, you start again from the last point of positive response and build on it.

6. Dramatic Words

'Hot words' is another brilliant conversational manipulation technique that is often used by glib conversationalists to hypnotize people. Our subconscious mind associates certain words and phrases with powerful emotions. There is a deep emotional or psychological significance linked to these words or phrases that almost always drives the subject into action.

Words such as "baby" "love" "trust" "assurance" and more incite a sense of warmth within the subject.

Once they respond to the hot words in a positive manner, you subtly begin to move to hypnotic words to first induce a state of relaxation, followed by a state of trance. For triggering a state of relaxation, you use words such as "relax." When you urge someone to relax, it triggers memories associated with relaxation such as lying on the beach or watching television. All the relaxation memories combine to make the person slip into a heightened state of relaxation.

This is followed by encouraging them to fixate their attention by using words such as "concentrate" or "focus." You have to emphasize words that essentially convey that a person should pass their regular conscious state and do things more unconsciously. Words such as "spontaneous" invoke those reactions or responses.

7. Amplifying Words

Much like hot or hypnotic words that are spoken to generate the desired reaction through the process of hypnosis, amplifying words increase or accelerate its pace. When you want your subject to perform a specific action, use words like "right now", "instantly" "immediately", "suddenly" etc. They create a rather dramatic effect or tension and a more powerful effect on the subject's unconscious mind, thus leading them to a response.

Chapter 2 Pros and Cons of Self-Discipline

Importance of Being Self-Disciplined

In this life, there are very many factors that contribute to a person's happiness and success. But in my opinion, there is one main factor that stands out from the rest, and that is self-discipline. Self-discipline brings with it sustainable and long-term effects in your life.

Persons with a high score in self-discipline do not let their choices or decisions to be impacted by their impulsive feelings and reactions. People who are disciplined always make rational choices in life, keeping in mind the possible result so that they do not get over upset or stressed if the outcomes are not as they had expected. Although many people know the benefits and the importance of being self-disciplined, only a few tend to put it into practice. Many are of the idea that being self-disciplined means one being harsh to themselves, to the extent of depriving themselves of happiness.

The advantages of being self-disciplined are as follows:

To be more efficient. People who are disciplined often make things easier for themselves to do their job. They put in place a structure or plan to be as much as productive as possible. This kind of people manages their little time well so as they can maximize their full capacity as an individual. Disciplined people also have an understanding of how to delegate tasks to other people who are perfect for the job, so that they can accomplish the tasks as a team.

To have a sense of direction in life. Being disciplined gives a person a sense of direction in their life. It mostly takes ample time and effort to accomplish goals that are in line. Students who have self-disciplined will more likely pass their exams compared to students who have a low level of self-discipline. Also, athletes who are more disciplined will tend to win in their respective races compared to those who are not disciplined. When you are disciplined, you can achieve whatever goal that you have set, and it can take you any place that you have ever dreamt of being. Self-discipline gives you a life that you dream of in which entertaining distractions and procrastination will never take you or give you.

Helps one to be more productive. If you are one person who has goals in life to be achieved, being more self-disciplined can make you very productive. People who have a high level of self-discipline do not allow procrastination to penetrate their lives. Removing distractions in one's life can be a little challenging for newly enlightened persons who want to become better in their lives. But as they keep the fire burning and practicing to remove all the distractions from their goals, they will learn how to meditate frequently, and within a short period, they will be more productive than ever. Most person who is very disciplined will not allow unproductive activities. Ensure that you do not perform things due to your impulsive reactions but make decisions or choices based on more important goals.

Brings more satisfaction in life. One gets satisfaction in life when they get what they want in life. If you want to assist other people in your society, put in on your to-do list! Do you desire to be a designer, architect, top class engineer? Always ensure that you put a plan in place. March forward and work your way through your plan to what you want to accomplish. Simple things like achieving a higher score in a test, understanding a subject in class, taking a bath, washing your clothes can make you feel more satisfied. The many stuff you perform, the more they will make you feel more satisfied.

Self-discipline will make you earn more respect. To be frank, not many people in the current generation have a high level of self-discipline. If you are one who has one, others will view you as some superhero that is capable of accomplishing many tasks in a very little amount of time. People who are disciplined know how to be accountable and responsible for whatever they do. This is what makes them be respected in society. In your society today, very few people dare to be scolded when something goes wrong. One who has a high level of self-control will shine in this kind of situation because they understand how to handle the situation appropriately, including the emotions.

Self-disciplined people have a high level of awareness. When you practice time management and work, they assist you in gaining a high level of awareness. These kinds of people know the factors that may challenge them from accomplishing their goals. Having a high level of awareness will make a person to easily notice factors that might help them accomplish their goals faster. In the corporate field, as you go up the hierarchy of management, a higher level of awareness is developed in you.

Being self-disciplined will make you live a happier life. Generally, when you are self-disciplined, you are happier in your life than those who are not. These types of people make wise choices in life and find ways of avoiding possible challenges that they may encounter. Self-discipline enhances your moods in times of trouble. When you are self-disciplined, you can relax and cope with different kinds of challenges in your life. Accomplishing goals is a measure of success that brings satisfaction, whose outcome is personal happiness.

Self-discipline improves your health. When you are productive, all you desire is to sustain a perfect state of health. You avoid losing the opportunity to do more tasks by just having a simple cough or, any other kind of illness. Control your desire to consume junk food and fast food and replace them with consuming a healthy diet. Through meditation, you can take care of your physical health as well as your mental health. Regular practicing of meditation enables you to de-clutter your mind with all kinds of mental garbage that distracts and drains you when doing your work. Meditation assists you to regulate your general being to have a more positive thought and outlook in your life and easily get rid of the negative thoughts that pop up in your mind frequently. When you are optimistic about everything in life, this will be one of the ultimate factors to your success in life.

Lack of Self-Discipline

Self-discipline shows up in every small thing that you do, be it at home or at your place of work. Some people ensure that they perform big deeds very well, but they ignore the small deeds. They do this only to impress some other people who do not know them well. But they disappoint and annoy those people who they work and live with; this shows that they do not value or care about the people they should show respect to.

When you ignore doing chores and duties, when you do not do what you say you would, when you do not turn up for appointments, when you do not look presentable, you manifest lack of self-discipline. Why don't you take responsibility for these daily obligations?

- Commitment. Your enthusiasm, commitment, and interest to a task determine the level to which you can be distracted. When your commitment is high, little things can't distract you, but if the task has no meaning to you, your attention is easily compromised or distracted. This proves that there is a powerful bond between self-discipline and commitment.

Lack of the ability to neglect, bypass, or control thoughts is lack of self-discipline.

- Attitude. This is because you do not believe in their importance. Why is it so? Why does a person go through a lot of difficulties to be sincere, considerate, clean, and trustworthy while another person seems to have a belief that these things are not so important? It is because of their attitude to themselves, life itself and to other people around them. The former has the belief that a person, including themselves, and other forms of life are worth spending their time, resources, energy and interest into. The person sees the sacredness of life. The latter has little regard for life and themselves.

All these relate to love. Because you have a love of life, you respect all aspects of life. You are taking time to nurture and appreciate life is no trouble. This should be a pleasure. You do this because you love life. It is no trouble at all. Self-discipline manifests itself from the willingness to nurture yourself, all other forms of life, and other people. Lack of self-discipline shows a little willingness to respect yourself or any other thing.

Factors Causing Lack or Poor Self-discipline

- Character. Weaknesses in your character can build poor self-discipline. Weaknesses such as

- Low level of courage,

- Low level of mental strength,

- Low level of your inner strength,

- Absence of self-love,

- Low interest in self-improvement in any aspect of your life,

- Lack of apathy,

- High levels of lust and greed,

- An aversion to hard work,

- Lack of love for God and other people,

- Lack of self-respect

- Shortage of responsibility

- An inability to neglect the temptation of self-indulgence and joy

If you love the thoughts, desires, emotions, and actions which harms you and other people more than you love life, your loved ones, God, yourself and other people be sure that you are destined for poor self-discipline. Ensure that each time you have an opportunity to choose what you do, you can perform something that will be helpful to other people, and also it can be spiritually uplifting. Or you can decide to do something selfish, obstructive, mean, destructive, and self-interested. The main motive behind your decision is either power or love. If you desire to show love, you will decide positive actions. If your desire is for power, your actions will always be negative.

Goals are not vital enough

If you set a goal which to you seems perfect, but you did not believe that the goal was necessary, or you do not see the goal as important enough for you to accomplish, then you will find it challenging to discipline yourself to complete the task and accomplish it. When your goals are not important, commitment is lacking. When there is importance in your goals in life, the level of commitment is high, and self-discipline is not that important. From that analogy, we can conclude that when a person lacks self-discipline, they also lack the commitment to their life itself. The person has no interest in life or has no proper understanding of life, its real purpose, and meaning.

Negative Impacts of Lack of Self Discipline

Low level of self-discipline in a person cause unhappiness; this is because all the aspects of happiness and all the techniques used to obtain happiness require self-discipline. With no self-discipline, little or no happiness is achieved. You will not restrain yourself from uttering or doing acts that will cause distress to loved ones or people who are around you and friends. For many people, this will result in misery for themselves.

Negative Effects include:

☐ Self-Destruction. Inadequate self-discipline means that you are going to be a victim of your passion for abnormal or excessive sexual indulgence, gambling, violence, gossip, eating unnecessarily, drugs, thrills, alcohol and other sensations and pleasures of the mind and the flesh. The challenges that these pleasures create in your life are too big and diverse to put up a list. Each time you allow these aberrations to tempt you, you are inviting suffering, grief, pain, misery, and misfortune in your life. The more you experience these negative aberrations in your life, the less fulfillment, freedom, love, contentment, and happiness you will enjoy. The choice is easy, but most of us find it difficult in making a wise decision.

☐ Lack of Responsibility. For people who find self-discipline unattainable, responsibility will be difficult for them. For you to accept responsibility, it means that you have to put aside other interest and desires when you have to attend to responsibilities. If your self-discipline is non-existent or slack, your preferences for many enjoyable actions will at times override your urge to keep the promises you made to others, and it will be disadvantaged by your ignorance attitude. This aspect may not cause worry to some people, but to those who are seeking a high level of respect from their fellow men, and for themselves, attending to their responsibilities is far too much important than any other thing.

It reaches even to the point that the loved ones are also put off. The self-discipline man has set a path for his life that even the loved ones can't understand and would not wish to be part of. The only option that the loved ones have been left with is for them to come together and save him from the situation. The actual situation is that the family members are more worried about themselves than they are about him. But does he have the courage and strength to stick to the choice that he had made which is going to cause a lot of crisis in his life? Does the man have the mental ability to withstand the many criticisms that are going to come his way? Many people are not. Many get to a point where the losses suffered are difficult to bear, and then the expected benefits of the new outcomes will have no positive impact on their life. This will lead to them weakening along the way, put aside their desires for self-improvement, and get themselves into a life full of apathy, boredom, and mediocrity.

Self-Inflicted Hardship. Every sorrow, sickness, hardship, pain, and unhappiness are direct consequences of your consciousness as manifested in your emotions, words, desires, actions, and thoughts. As already explained and shown that your desires cause most of your problems. By you stopping to have desires, by you not wanting anything or expecting any particular results, and by you reducing the impacts of your emotions on yourself, you are going to rid yourself of many reasons that cause your problems.

Emotions and passions destroy self-confidence. Each time you decide to perform a task, set a goal, and make up your mind on your course action, your emotions and desires intervene and point out a list of more enjoyable, interesting things for you to do instead. Only people with a high level of mental toughness, self-discipline and courage can neglect desires for the more relaxing and enjoyable activities, for them to choose to pay attention and focus their energy to the task they are required to accomplish their life desires. As soon as you submit to your emotions and your passion, you allow yourself down and betray yourself. Deep down, you know this, and your self-respect and self-esteem plummet. Your self-confidence depends on your self-belief because you need faith in your capability to finish the tasks you set yourself. Whenever you surrender to your desires, you lose a little self-confidence.

Self Interest. Although, when it comes to personal growth, you put a lot of emphasis on yourself, it is not for your gain in a material sense or for you to have more influence over other people, rather it is for you to become more, helpful, sincere, loving, and kind as a person. You apply self-discipline in the hope that you develop the noble human traits. A person who put their positive energy to getting more power, material goods, thrills and influence out of their actions in life for their self-interest tend to show no or less concern for anyone else apart from themselves. All you need is self-discipline for you to think about the welfare of others around you in all that you do. This explains why a little percentage of the world's population practices self-discipline.

Desires. Your desires make up the source of many of the problems you experience in your life. Many will argue that accomplishing their desires are their core source of fulfillment, happiness, and contentment. Even though some desires are positive, a large percent is negative and may cause more negative karma as well as causing more conflict, worry, and problems. Self-discipline helps you to overcome your yearning to satisfy your harmful desires.

Complacency. Your lack of self-discipline makes you avoid some responsibilities, chores, and duties that you should be doing at some specific time. You sometimes do not experience disadvantage or retribution because of your poor self-discipline; you tend to be complacent and choose that some tasks do not have to be done anyway. At this point, procrastination becomes part of you. You should know that in the long run, complacency and ignorance will always come back to hurt you.

Procrastination. You will realize that with no doubt that lack of self-discipline is a major contributing factor in procrastination.

A person who cannot make themselves to do what should be done will procrastinate when a task they have an aversion to present itself. If you have a certain level of self-discipline, you will act in the task given immediately. People with less self-discipline will procrastinate as long as they can without them upsetting anyone else that much.

Relaxation. Lack of self-discipline hinders you from full relaxation. It may seek not of any importance for you to have self-discipline for you to relax, but the opposite is true. Self-discipline implies that you are rigid, firm, and tense. These attitudes are counterproductive for relaxation. When one is relaxing, he/she should be able to dismiss desires, thoughts, and emotions from your consciousness and clear your mind of any worries or negative thoughts, attitudes, and concerns. If you are not able to accomplish this, relaxation will not be possible. You will require mental and emotional self-discipline.

Poor Health. Most of the health disorders are the outcome of karma. However, this should not be a reason by those who have a low level of self-discipline for them not to practice methods that enhance a healthier body.

Poor performance with Goals. When a person has no actual understanding of the purpose and meaning of life, they find it difficult to find a convincing reason why they do many of the things that occupy most of their time and consume all their positive energy. When it comes to goal setting, what motivates them to tend to be self-gratification and self-interest. Self-interest and self-gratification will tend to lose their appeal quickly, and the commitment needed to pursue the goals will quickly disintegrate.

Chapter 3 Why Constraints are Necessary

Constraints and self-discipline. It is easy to tell ourselves that we don't have the time for the energy or the skills or the connections to accomplish the goals we set for ourselves.

These self-imposed constraints, real or otherwise, can keep you in an endless loop of wanting something, feeling that the universe is conspiring against you, and preventing you from obtaining what you want.

However, there is a better way to look at this.

View the constraint as something good. How can not having something help us become better at a skill? Here is why, it forces you to develop the skill that would otherwise go undeveloped, because you did not have that constraint in place in the first place.

What this means is simple.

If, for example, you do not like getting up early but you want to develop the habit of getting up early. You have now forced yourself into a time constraint giving you the option of waking up and starting your day earlier than before.

I recommend trying things in very small chunks and I also recommend making whatever goal you want to accomplish very specific.

Let's stay with our example. You want to establish the habit of getting up earlier, say 6 AM every day so that you are not rushing out the door to get to work and you can have time to either read, meditate, write, whatever it is you are missing out on because you are starting your day behind the eight ball and late.

By giving yourself just one week, you are giving yourself the best chance of obtaining the goal of getting up earlier with less chance of failure.

Also by committing to one week, if that particular goal is not right for you, you can stick it out for seven days and then decide that you may want to try something else.

Perhaps it is a specific skill you want to develop and not a behavior.

I know I wanted to develop the skill of writing daily. What does it take to become a better writer? Very simple but not easy. One needs to write consistently. If I get up first thing in the morning and write down whatever it is, I decide to write that morning, generally it is just a brain dump, I find that writing other things is much easier.

By writing daily, the ability becomes much more effortless and second nature, which makes me extend my goal. So now instead of seven days. I will commit to two weeks and then three and then four until it is a daily habit and something as natural to me as brushing my teeth.

James Clear says focus on something you want to develop. Make it very specific. For example, you cannot tell yourself you want to be good at business or communication.

Both of these skills are broad topics they are not skills per se. They are areas to master and very broad and general.

Instead, do this, tell yourself, 'I want to make 25 phone calls every morning before 8 AM to potential clients.'

It does not matter if every call hangs up on you. You are developing the necessary skill to become better at that facet of business.

You can then carry that over into other areas of your business, such as becoming better at business accounting or bookkeeping so that you know where your money is going. It can go on and on like this. As you develop each skill you get stronger in your field.

Another example would be to say I want to be good at communication. What does that mean exactly? Communication can range from delivered speeches to a crowd of people all the way down to a text message from a friend saying they are running late.

What you do instead is say I want to sit down with my spouse every Wednesday at 8 o'clock after the kids have gone to bed and discuss items we don't normally get to discuss because we are so busy.

This will improve the relationship as well as improve your communication skills. You can even take it one step further and say during that time, I am going to be a better listener and truly empathize with my partner so that he or she can see that I truly understand where he or she is coming from.

You can then extend this open communication skill into other areas as well such as work, where you may want to say, I want to discuss this project with my boss in a positive and constructive manner. Perhaps this is a touchy area and you and your boss have clashed over it in the past.

Make it a game. Look at the constraints you have as obstacles in a videogame that you need to get past. Mario, of the popular Nintendo games does not complain as he makes his way through the various constraints placed in front of him as he tries to rescue the princess. No, he takes each one and overcomes them as they pop up. You can do the same. You won't see it as something holding you back and it will make it much funner for you to attempt. You are simply playing within the rules of the game now. By reframing the problem into this light. You have shown yourself that you can accomplish goals in the process of developing self-discipline becomes much more fun.

There are only three things that can be manipulated to develop the specific skill you want to develop time, resources, and your environment.

Let's take a look at each constraint and see how we can make them work for us.

Time, this resource is usually everyone's biggest obstacle. Let's say your boss gives you a project that is due in one month. The old way of doing it, as Albert Einstein says, would be to allow the time given and use up every second of it until it is due within 30 days.

How about giving yourself a self-imposed deadline of seven days? See what happens, I think you will be surprised.

Resources, if you travel pack light, put everything you will take on that trip into one carry-on bag or a backpack. This forces you to break it down into the bare essentials. It also frees you up considerably to be able to move in a much more relaxed way because you are not worried about your luggage being lost or having to carry heavy suitcases everywhere you go.

Your environment. Let's say you work with access to the Internet. It can be a giant time suck and is limitless in its ability to induce dopamine rushes of intense euphoria as you search and forage for newer and better information.

How about turning it off and not checking it at all while you are engaged in whatever project you happen to be doing, whether it be at work or at home? Make your office a no-go zone for technology other than say your word processing or spreadsheet document.

What do you want to become good at? What is important to you and to your career to turn it into the life that you want developed?

Sit down and really think about these things. Give them deep thought and as you design your tasks and projects use them as a way to create self-discipline in your life.

Is it easy? Absolutely not. But using this as a reframing tool. It gives you the ability to see things in a much more positive light. View your constraints with new eyes. View them as helping you not holding you back.

Chapter 4 How to Build Self-Discipline

Building self-discipline is not as hard as your mind might have been conditioned to believe, though it will not come without some efforts and commitment. Here are some tested and trusted techniques you can adopt to help you build and maintain self-discipline.

Understand Where You Draw Inspiration from and What Turns Your Light Off

You have things that trigger your weaknesses and things that feed your major strengths. Discovering things that bring out the best in you and the things that bring your weakest points to the fore will go a long way toward building your self-discipline. This means you must commit some time to learn more about yourself. Building self-discipline boils down to overcoming your strongest negative urges, cravings, and desires.

Set a Goal

Every great achievement in life begins with setting a feasible goal. By "feasible," I mean a goal that can be achieved within the deadline, all things being fair. In setting a goal to become more self-disciplined, you must put several factors into consideration, such as your most dominant traits, your habits, your major strengths, your weaknesses, things you have become addicted to, things you would want to change in your life, etc. Your goal should have a date for beginning your efforts to increase your level of self-discipline and a date by which you must have improved your level of self-discipline drastically.

Have a Plan

A goal might not be enough to take you to where you are going if you do not have a plan for how to get there. A goal tells you where you wish to go and when you wish to get there, but a plan helps you know the right path to take in order to arrive at your destination on time. Your plan should be detailed and tabulated. Your plan should involve daily activities you can engage in to help you become more self-disciplined.

Have Your Goal and Your Plan Written Down

Write down your goals and plans and place them where you can see them several times a day. You can post them on the walls of your room to enable you to get a glimpse of them the moment you rise in the morning and before you sleep at night. This constant reminding will help you keep the goal fresh and stay focused while on your self-discipline building project.

Start with Baby Steps

When it comes to how to build self-discipline, it is important to begin with simple baby steps you can easily learn to practice and move on to more complex steps as you record improvements. Building your self-discipline, like every other important lifestyle change in life, will not happen overnight.

Deny Yourself Certain Pleasures

Denying yourself certain pleasures will enable you to learn how to be in control of your life. It is all about practicing and mastering self-restraint. Force yourself to quit every old habit that hinders you from becoming a better you. Develop a deep hatred for things that distract you from pursuing your goals, such as TV addiction and excessive intake of drugs and alcohol. Holding on to any of these things that give you momentary pleasures will hinder you from amounting to anything meaningful in life. Find other ways to keep yourself occupied such as reading, working on a new business plan, volunteering in a community project, taking part in religious meetings, etc.

Get Rid of All Negative Habits

You can't be talking about becoming self-disciplined when you have not dealt with habits that are clear manifestations of your indiscipline. Getting rid of some negative habits won't be easy at all, because old habits die hard. However, with the right efforts and commitments, you can change any habit. One way to get rid of negative habits is to think about the habit thoroughly, weighing its benefits against its disadvantages. If possible, do some researches about that particular habit to enable you to get more facts about it, and then imagine what life could look like without those negative habits and find a constructive habit to replace the unconstructive habit.

Dump Your Negative Friends

The truth about self-discipline and the relationships you keep is that you can never become self-disciplined if you keep hanging out with the wrong crowd. If your circle of friends is made up of a bunch of undisciplined people, it will take a sort of a miracle for you to manage to have any self-discipline. Having friends who do not value self-discipline means you will always find yourself where negative behaviors are being exhibited. To build your self-discipline, it is important you get rid of friends that do not encourage you in your efforts to build discipline.

Change Environments

Nothing affects your habits and the habits of your children more than the environment you spend most of your daily time in. If you live in a city or district where good manners and habits have been thrown to the swine, it will be hard for you to cultivate any good habits toward becoming more self-disciplined. If you want to become a more self-disciplined person, perhaps you could start considering moving to a new home. Find a better neighborhood where people still have enough conscience not to engage in stomach-churning behaviors. Change your church, school, gym, etc., to help you meet people who value good morals and positive habits like you do.

Adopt New Daily Habits

Daily good habits are an excellent start to build self-discipline. Runners, for example, have to wake up every day, have breakfast on time, and go jogging at a specific time for a pre-defined amount of time. You can, with enough willpower, create good habits.

PERSEVERE

Don't make the mistake of thinking you are now disciplined because you have been able to deal with bad habits such as addictions to harmful drugs and alcohol, overfeeding, arrogance, financial recklessness, infidelity, insincerity, etc. Some of these old habits will often want to return to you after a while. Whenever you fall into any of these ditched habits as a result of momentary weakness, you must make sure you get up and keep moving without looking back. Falling is normal on any success journey — it is staying down that makes you a failure. When you fall, make sure you get up faster than you fell.

Find Some Role Models

When talking about role models, I don't mean the music and movie stars you probably admire for their fashion sense. By "role models," I mean people whose life stories can inspire you to become a better you and reach for greater heights in life. Find people who have been through where and what you are going through, then learn how they overcame their challenges and strategies they adopted to win their life battles.

Whatever It Takes, Make Sure You Leave No Tasks Unaccomplished

One sure thing that helps you build self-discipline is to ensure you complete your current tasks before moving to other tasks. No matter the goal you are working towards — be it losing those unwanted pounds of flesh; starting that new business; learning how to be an expert in music, sports, drawing, or painting; or becoming a better politician — if you are on any of these tasks, you must follow through with the training and learning. It makes you more prepared for becoming the best in what you do.

Chapter 5 Self-Discipline Strategies

Now that you have worked through the power of habits and the power of productivity, it is time to start digging into some strategies that are specifically going to help you with your self-discipline! The strategies that are going to help you with your self-discipline are ones that teach you how you can begin to have more control over yourself and over your results in life, which makes them extremely valuable. You are going to want to start learning how you can implement every single one of these strategies into your life if you want to become self-disciplined like the successful businessmen that you follow and aspire to be like. If you truly want to tap into their secrets, the secret is that they do every single one of these strategies, plus all of the others listed in this book, and it is through that which they are able to experience success in their lives. These are the secret behaviors that they learned, not that they were born with, that allow them to excel beyond the rest and truly set themselves apart. It is by engaging in these strategies that they are able to really master self-discipline and increase their success tenfold and beyond.

How Self-Discipline Strategies Help

Self-discipline strategies help by giving you opportunities to really learn how to gain control over yourself and over your mind so that you can achieve your goals in life. If you want to accelerate in life and really develop to a higher level of success, then practicing self-discipline strategies is necessary so that you can grow beyond where you presently are at. Self-discipline strategies help you embody the habits and behaviors of someone who is achieving next-level success, so it is highly important that you learn about what these are and how they work.

Every single strategy that you are going to learn about is going to help you either by increasing your self-awareness or by helping you learn how to override your emotional brain and gain control over your mind. This way, despite the habitual protest that may arise from your mind, you are able to continue developing your skills and moving beyond obstacles so that you can attain the level of success that you desire. For anyone who wants to get ahead in life, this is necessary. These are the very strategies that make the difference between working for minimum wage at a stressful job and hating your day-to-day life and working for a high-value pay at an enjoyable career and loving your life. These are the difference between being in low-quality relationships that you dread partaking in and being in thriving relationships that you love to take part in and nourish so that they can continue to grow and flourish. These strategies are the difference between living a miserable life that brings you stress and disappointment in many different ways and living a life that you are proud of and that you can feel confident showing up for every single day.

Developing a Growth Mindset

As I mentioned previously, a growth mindset can be powerful in developing your productivity, as well as increasing your self-discipline. A growth mindset is essentially a name for someone who is open-minded and willing to learn and search for solutions to that which they are going through in life. If you have a growth mentality, you are focused on developing your skills and finding ways to move through obstacles that may present themselves along your journey so that you can continue to develop along your path. This way, regardless of what you are up against in life, you are willing to find a way to grow through it and advance toward your goals.

Developing a growth mindset requires you to begin learning how to intentionally open your mind so that you can keep finding your way to your next stage of growth. There are many strategies that you can use that help you develop your growth mindset, but I am going to share the best ones with you, starting with learning to shift how you view challenges in your life. The natural way for many people to perceive challenges in their life is as an incredibly difficult obstacle. Often, their thought process stops there and they never put in the effort to look into how a challenge can be perceived or overcome, but instead, they see it as something that can bring all of their progress and effort to a full stop. If you want to change your entire mindset in one just one move, learn how to develop a mindset that allows you to see every challenge as an opportunity to grow and learn new skills. This way, you begin to develop curiosity and excitement around challenges, rather than fears and uncertainty. As you continue to develop this, you will find that you are better able to overcome obstacles in your life and that rather than procrastinating and feeling overwhelmed or incapable, you begin to feel like there is always a solution for you.

Another big way that you can develop a growth mindset is to stop seeking approval and validation from external sources. Many times, when we are heavily focused on pleasing those around us, we find that we are constantly focused on their reactions and opinions about what we are doing rather than our own. This can lead to a close-mindedness that stems from you attempting to think in terms of what would make someone else happy, rather than what would make you happy. In the end, you may find yourself avoiding solutions or certain types of growth because you are afraid that other people will not approve of or validate you if you pursue this path, even if it feels like the right path for you.

If seeking validation and approval is important to you, or does influence you in any way, begin learning how you can portray criticism as a positive thing in your life, rather than a negative. So, rather than believing that every time someone criticizes you it automatically means that you are bad or incapable, begin to see this as an opportunity to find new ways to grow. In some cases, criticism will mean virtually nothing because you are already satisfied with where you have grown to, but in others, you might need to allow yourself to find growth opportunities in what someone has said to you. So, rather than seeing criticism as some form of punishment or reprimanding for doing something wrong, see it as an opportunity to do even better next time so that you can further improve on your skill.

A great way to get to the point where you can see criticism as constructive or positive is by allowing yourself to see that you are imperfect and to focus on your growth rather than your perfection. When you accept from the start that you are not perfect and you begin focusing on how you can improve and grow rather than how you can be perfect everything changes. This way, you are no longer focusing on perfection and feeling ashamed when people offer constructive criticism. Instead, you are grateful for the advice and you apply this to your existing knowledge so that you can continually improve and work toward developing better skills over time.

Lastly, if you really want to develop a growth mindset, focus on growth and effort over speed and talent. The more you truly make the growth the goal and focus on the effort that you are putting into everything that you do, the more you are going to be able to continue developing and growing over time. This stops you from trying to rush the process, speed to the finish line, or have the best talent of anyone. Instead, you are so immersed with and engaged in the growing process that you are genuinely enjoying yourself and all that growth has to offer you, thus helping you anchor in a growth mindset.

Finding Your Personal Mission

When it comes to developing self-discipline, nothing will serve you more than having a strong set of values that are guiding you toward what it is that you truly want in life. When you know what it is that you desire and exactly what you are working toward, developing your self-discipline becomes easier because you have a clear goal for what it is that you desire to achieve in your life. This way, you are able to continue motivating yourself to move forward because you are on a personal mission that keeps you feeling committed to your work for the long haul.

Finding your personal mission if you have not already is not as hard as you may think. Chances are, you have already found your personal mission, yet you have never actually identified it because it comes so naturally to you and it may not stand out as anything significant or special. In many cases, people find that their personal missions are things that they have already been into or committed to for their life yet they are so used to being committed to this mission that it does not stand out to them. For that reason, finding your personal mission is typically more focused on reflection than it is on actually going out and finding something to be committed to.

A great way to begin discovering what your personal mission is would be to start asking yourself reflective questions that help you reflect on what it is that you have already created so that you can discover what truly matters to you, and what you value in this life. You can start by asking yourself easier questions like, what makes you smile. What is your favorite thing to do? And what do you lose track of time doing? You can also ask yourself questions such as who inspires you and who shows up in this world in a way that you are inspired by? Asking yourself these types of questions helps you discover what you are already interested in and what is interesting enough to captivate your attention even when other people are engaging in that behavior.

Another series of questions you can ask yourself revolve around your personal mastery. Questions like, what are you naturally good at? What could you easily teach? And what can you see yourself regretting if you did not fully engage in it in this lifetime? These questions help you identify what you are already good at, where your natural talents lie, and how you can begin finding the things that truly stand out to you in life. When you begin purposefully engaging in these practices, you will find that your natural passion and interest in them are ignited as you begin digging even deeper into what truly matters to you.

If you really want to validate whether or not something is your life mission, you can do a great visualization practice that will help you determine what truly matters to you and what you genuinely want to do with your life. The visualization is simple: imagine you are 90 years old and you are sitting on your rocking chair on the patio drinking iced water and looking out into the neighborhood as people walk by. You are happy and at peace, and you feel that you have had a wonderful life and you are grateful for all that you contributed to the world in the ways that you contributed. You achieved and acquired everything that mattered to you, you cultivated powerful relationships with people you loved, and you have developed in a way that is beyond your wildest dreams. Now, reflect back on your life that got you to 90 years old. What did you do? What was your mission? How did you contribute to the world that also contributed to your personal joy, happiness, and feelings of achievement? This is a great visualization tool to use to help you look into the bigger picture and see what truly matters to you and what you genuinely want to become known for in this lifetime.

You can also begin to ask yourself questions such as, based on your natural talents and gifts, what type of meaningful work could you serve that would light your heart up and leave you feeling purposeful and meaningful in this lifetime? For people who are not fully aware of how their gifts can translate into a meaningful mission, this is a great opportunity to develop a meaningful personal mission from your gifts and turn them into something special.

Once you have identified what your mission ought to be, you can go ahead and write your personal mission statement. Your personal mission statement is a single sentence that summarizes what your primary goal or focus is in life, allowing you to have a very clear sense of direction toward what you want to create in this lifetime. Some examples of great personal mission statements include:

- Denise Morrison of the Campbell Soup Company: "To serve as a leader, live a balanced life, and apply ethical principles to make a significant difference."
- Oprah Winfrey of the Oprah Winfrey Network (OWN): "To be a teacher, and to be known for inspiring my students to be more than they thought they could be."
- Richard Branson of The Virgin Group: "To have fun in (my) journey through life and learn from (my) mistakes."

As you can see, anything can be a mission statement, as long as it is personal to you. Because your mission statement is relevant only to your personal journey in life, creating your mission statement can be personal as well. Remember, make your personal mission statement *personal,* because the only person it needs to inspire and motivate is *you.*

How to Set Effective Goals

Setting effective goals is a great way to increase your self-discipline. When you have set effective goals, advancing toward your desired outcomes is easier because you have planned a clear-cut path toward what it is that you desire to achieve. Although plans do not always go as we thought they would, identifying at least a basic path forward is a great opportunity for you to begin moving forward with anything that you are trying to achieve in life. When you set effective goals, you give your mind a sense of safety by showing yourself that there is a clear path for you to be talking and that it leads you to where you want to go. For people who find themselves engaging in procrastination due to uncertainty, this leads to them resolving the primary reason why they are not advancing so that they can begin to proceed toward their goals with confidence.

You have likely heard of the term "SMART" goals at least a thousand times, so rather than teaching you what you already know, I want to give you a refresher on what this acronym means and how you can take it a step further to really create the best goals that keep you on track. To remind you, SMART goals stand for goals that are: specific, measurable, attainable, realistic, and timely. Having SMART goals allows you to have goals that are clearly defined so that you can begin to walk a path forward toward what it is that you desire. The thing about SMART goals is that, while they define a clear outcome, they do not always require you to define a clear path. Ideally, if you have made a SMART goal because it is *measurable*, a path can certainly be made, so putting in the effort to actually make one is important. This is where you can go from making SMART goals to making genius goals if you know what I mean!

Setting an effective SMART goal with a path starts with identifying exactly what it is that you are working toward, or what your SMART goal has outlined for you. Then, you want to start working backward to create a custom pathway that will successfully lead you toward the outcome that you desire to achieve in life. Start with the goal, and then ask yourself what milestone will be accomplished right before you achieve that goal that allows you to know that you are almost there. Continue working backward down your list of milestones until you get to where you are at right now, which will connect you from here to your goal. This way, you have successfully identified a path that is going to set you up for success.

Once you have identified what your pathway is going to be for your goal, it is important that you develop the right mindset around your pathway so that you can maintain a growth mindset that keeps you moving forward toward your goal. A great way to do this is to immediately set the intention that you are going to use this path as your path forward until you are shown a better way. What this means is that you are going to assume that you have outlined the best way forward with the knowledge that you presently have in your possession, but if you were to come across knowledge that showed you a better way in the future, you would use that. Keeping this mindset ensures that you stay committed to your path by committing to taking action right now, while also keeping you flexible in what you may learn along the way. This protects you against two different kinds of stubbornness: the type that stems from feeling like your plan is not good enough, and the type that stems from being unwilling to change your plan.

If you develop the type of stubbornness that leads you to believe that your plan is not good enough, you may begin practicing procrastination by assuming that you are not going to make enough growth through your current path to get you anywhere. Of course, this leads to you staying still and never discovering the knowledge that you would need to adjust your plan should that be necessary, which ultimately leads to you letting yourself down because you are unwilling to advance down the path that will lead you to success.

If you develop the type of stubbornness that has you close-minded to the idea of shifting your plan when you learn new information, you may end up missing your goal entirely or taking forever to get there because you were too stubborn to adapt. In this situation, you let your ego tell you that you know all and that your plan is the best plan and no one and nothing could possibly improve on it, which can lead to you taking significantly longer to get to where you want to go. In this case, you may end up wasting time and a significant amount of resources because you were too stubborn to trust the new information that you learned about and turn it into a strategy to advance faster. In either case, if you adopt stubbornness, you lose. So, at the end of the day, developing an effective goal *and* embodying a growth mindset are two powerful tools to help you continually move forward if you want to grow your self-discipline and make progress toward your goals in life.

Understanding Your Personal "Why"

In addition to having a personal mission statement, which is your end goal, you should also work toward developing a personal why. Your why is what is going to encourage you to make the plan to achieve your goal in the first place and to follow that plan every step of the way. Your why is what truly gives meaning to your goal so that you can stay committed and continually work toward that with intention and a significant sense of personal power.

Developing your personal why is not unlike developing a purpose for your business or your business goals if you are an entrepreneur. It starts by identifying what your purpose is and identifying what the beliefs are that are driving you forward in achieving the goal that you have set out to achieve. A great way to understand what your why is meant to answer is to ask yourself these questions:

- "WHY are you alive right now?"

- "WHY were you inspired to get out of bed this morning?"
- "WHY should people care about this?"

These types of question help give your personal mission meaning and significance, and while it does not need to be developed to please anyone else, considering how you justify the significance of your personal mission can help you identify why it matters. Your why statement sets you apart from everyone else and gives you a strong motivation to move ahead in life and steadily work toward what you want to achieve. When you nurture your why and you keep it personal and relevant to yourself, you make it easier for you to really keep yourself driven and moving forward toward your goals in life, so it is imperative that you pick something that is more than just a little important to you. For example, if you like the idea of making money but you love the idea of saving animals, then your why should be serving animals, not making money. Pick something that completely lights you up.

When it comes to your why statement, you can certainly pick more than one motivator, but you should avoid picking more than three. Although there may be many things motivating you, keeping your why statement simple with one to three primary motivators helps you really stay focused on what is driving you. This way, these motivators are significant and they carry larger value, rather than being diluted by the fact that there are so many that you are paying attention to and working toward. If you have too many motivators in your why statement, you may find that you are not fully driven by any of them because none of them are truly that significant to you. Be honest with what drives you and make that your primary driver. As well, remember that this is private and only for you, so do not feel like your why has to sound significant or profound to anyone else, as the only person it needs to sound significant or profound to is yourself.

Chapter 6 Immerse Yourself in the Culture of Self-Discipline

The first people who have introduced us to the concept of discipline were our parents. In the absence of parents, we had father and mother figures in the form of mentors, older relatives, or older peers. The way we learn about the world is through the world itself, and through the people around us. We model ourselves based on them. Discipline starts at home. You cannot help but become disciplined yourself when disciplined people surround you. A perfect example of the culture of self-discipline is the Special Operations Units.

All the men in the military follow a code. Their training, governing systems and operating procedures were all developed while considering the military code. Soldiers who show dedication in practicing this code may advance to more elite branches of the military. This separates them from other members of the armed forces and gives credit to their skills and knowledge of their craft.

When they advance to these elite branches or special forces, the types of people that they spend time with also change. Their peers in the special forces are those who are also as dedicated in their craft and in keeping their country safe.

The presence of their peers reminds the member of this branch every day of the special force's code that they live by. If everybody in the group works out regularly, it will compel the newer members to do the same. If all the members have excellent skills, the new members need to push themselves to improve their own skills. These are just some of the effects of being around people with excellent self-discipline.

Surround Yourself with Disciplined People

When developing your own self-discipline, you need to surround yourself with people who have the same goals and aspirations as you. It is even better if you can find people who are very dedicated to their work. By surrounding yourself with these types of people, you will have someone with which you can compare yourself. If you are competitive by nature, having people around you who are good at what they do can ignite your competitive spirit in you. This can be a great source of extrinsic motivation.

In your job, for example, you can look for the top performers in your office. Take the time to talk with them when they are free. If they are busy all the time, you can invite them to lunch. You can also go to the social events where the people you look up to go. If you are in the office, you can also observe them when they are working and look for what separates them from the pack.

Your goal is to spend time with them and learn about how they perform so well. It is important, also to humble yourself in the presence of more disciplined people. A child who is learning a new skill puts himself in an inferior position in order to learn faster. No self-obsessed conceited man with a superiority complex can begin to understand true self-discipline if he thinks that he is already better than everyone around him. In surrounding yourself with highly disciplined people, you must put yourself in the inferior position, like a child, in order to learn their ways and quickly become like them.

Developing Your Own Group of Highly Disciplined People

In developing all the habits discussed in this book, you will need two important components:

1. Find self-improvement buddies

Before you do any of the habits suggested in this chapter, you need to look for a person who will help you become accountable for your commitments. You need a buddy who will keep an eye on you and make sure that you do the tasks properly and on time. Ideally, you need to find a buddy who also wants to develop his own self-discipline. If you have a friend undergoing the same difficulties as you, you will have a better chance of convincing yourself to be committed to the tasks required by this book.

It is better if your buddy is ruthless in reminding you about your tasks. He should not allow you to be weak. He should be able to shout in your face when you stay in bed too long in the morning. You should do the same for him. Your standards should be high when critiquing each other's actions. You can start with a co-worker or a roommate. If you have siblings, you can also show them this book.

2. Set punishments for failure or unfinished tasks

In the military, men complete the tasks that they need to do because they do not have a choice. The drill sergeants remove the idea of having a choice. Either you do what they want, or you quit the military life because you are too weak. This prepares the soldiers for the active service. When they are in the field, they are accustomed to following orders, and they do not question the decisions decided upon by their superiors. In this kind of practice, you are able to learn the value of trusting your superiors. If you are capable of following your superiors, you will be able to set your own rules soon and follow them by yourself.

Just like in the military, the punishment that you set should be physical in nature. Push-ups and squats are the common punishments among the basic training of all the branches of the military. You could also think of undesirable chores like cleaning the backyard or the toilet and doing your buddy's laundry.

Now that you have the necessary requirements for developing special forces culture, you need to learn the habits that you need to integrate into your life. These habits are designed to make you disciplined from your waking to your sleeping hour.

Chapter 7 Create Discipline and Build Your Own Daily Routine

Increment Your Willpower with Meditation

Regardless of whether it's a sparkling recognition, a rocking body, an eye-popping financial balance. It may be a regular satisfying vocation, a change the world business, picture impeccable wellbeing, or some other objective — you should prepare yourself to do the things you don't generally want to do however know you need to'."

Would it be appropriate for me to remain stuck to the love seat throughout the evening or hit the rec center? Would it suffice if Netflix (for one more night) or make some new companions at that neighborhood Meetup?

Would it be advisable for me to proceed with my unlimited internet-based life scroll or (at last) begin on figuring out how to code? Would it be a good idea for me to fund this fresh out of the plastic new vehicle or pay money for something more established?

Would it be advisable for me to enjoy this brownie or hold off until I have accomplished shoreline body status? Would it be advisable for me to play an additional two hours of Fortnight or kick things off on my virtuoso startup thought?

Without the self-restraint to put in the "hard yards" today, the fantasy of a superior tomorrow will consistently be only that — a fantasy. Fortunately, we aren't brought into the world with a set measure of determination. All the incredible ones had it; you can do it as well.

Before we disclose to you the key to amplifying your internal quality, it's critical to comprehend what makes the "high accomplishing" cerebrum so remarkable.

Why Meditation Is The Secret To Building Willpower

Alright, changing my life is unquestionably conceivable. I am much obliged to you for opening my eyes to that. However, likely not going to' occur. Why? Since shortcoming rules my present reality. What's the key to hitting my determination switch?

To recover the light in your eyes, you have to sustain your inner world. Also, the ideal approach to do that? Reflection. Understanding reflection's fleeting effect on discretion begins with that enormous delightful arch sitting on your (destined to be) etched shoulders. Here's how it works:

Intending to pinpoint determination's place of residence (in mind), Caltech neuroscientists (Hare et al) had 37 calorie counters rate 50 pictures of sustenance on their degree of "wonderfulness" and "fitness." The weight watchers were then snared to cerebrum imaging innovation and educated to pick between nourishment they evaluated as "unbiased" (for example wheat diminishes, granola) and either a "scrumptious" sustenance (for example cheddar cake, chocolate) or "solid" sustenance (for example broccoli, celery). What did they find?

At the point when the weight watchers made wellbeing driven (as opposed to taste-driven) nourishment decisions, an area of their cerebrum called the "dorsolateral prefrontal cortex" (DL-PFC) lit up like the sky on fourth of July. I'm not catching this' meaning? This heap of cells covered profound behind the temple is self-control's home in the cerebrum.

While contemplation's "internal world" bulletproofing advantages have been known and expounded on for a very long time, seeing it affirmed (utilizing the most recent logical gadgetry, no less) is a different situation. For those of us looking for a superior life (aren't we as a whole!), this is excellent news.

Through the unbelievable intensity of neuroplasticity, reflection causes you "do the things you don't generally wanna' do however know you need.' From practicing more to eating better, to kicking habit, to adapting new aptitudes, to accomplishing your dream(s), contemplation's "inward quality" amplification improves existence on all phases.

Self-restraint Positive Affirmations

I will sit tight for remuneration.

I invest the energy, exertion, and control required to accomplish my objectives.

I utilize conscious thought when settling on decisions in regards to my time.

I ceaselessly take activities that help my most astounding potential.

I let all desires go. My objectives are my inspiration.

I am glad for the center I bring to my life.

I use my assets as well as could be expected.

I respect my most astounding goals.

I can turn into the best in my field.

I let all diversions go. My complete consideration is toward carrying on with my best life.

Utilizing Visualization for Self-Development

Perceptions, or seeing yourself in a specific circumstance, has helped numerous individuals throughout the years to develop an uplifting outlook. Through perception, one can rationally go anyplace and utilize the implementers by asserting what they need from life, to arrive. Insistences are announcements that we can make that give us inward help. It is our method for affirming what we plan to do. Attestations give us affirmations that confirm our expectations through the explanations that we make. It fabricates support so one can stand firm while moving in the direction of a superior future.

At the point when a few people consider perception, they begin to build up this mental picture in their brain of somebody that has an issue with fantasizing or daydreaming. A few people even believe that representations are predictions. In opposition to these convictions, perceptions are mental pictures that we make, which impact our fantasies and perspective.

Utilizing our perception and affirmatives, we can push toward a positive future while building up the internal identity. Self-improvement begins in the belly and conveys forward over an incredible span. All through this stage, one learns, while picking up information from encounters and occasions seen by the eye. Probably the ideal approaches to support representation while elevating our talent to utilize affirmatives is through reflection or yoga.

Contemplation will help you with putting your brain in a period where you can picture the self in a scene while you trust you need to be. Through guided unwinding strategies, it will wind up simpler with each mental picture you create, since you will begin thinking positive. You have to create positive intuition to profit by affirmatives. What, is it workable for somebody to picture and assert while going from start to finish of the self-improvement stages? Is it conceivable to work throughout self-improvement by utilizing perceptions and certifications?

Indeed, it is conceivable to utilize visuals and affirmatives to control through self-advancement. Since self-advancement is a procedure, it is always decent to have our psychological limit and capacities helping us en route. We need backing and help from others. It is decent to have companions that offer comparable characteristics as yourself. It gives you motivation since you don't wind up acting as though you are in an immense world without anyone else's input. Having individuals around you with parallel interests is a part of self-improvement.

Other human formative abilities are additionally helpful. We gain from internal identity. The internal identity is our executive. Therefore, the man in control that helps us through the self-development stage in spite of that we may slack in territories. A great many people don't perceive that usually, we as a whole create to specific levels. Since, impacts factor into our advancement, we see that it could make issues. Issues could grow, for example, unfortunate propensities, practices, thinking, etc. This is regularly obvious when we partner with individuals that think negative and mirror their intuition on us. Our practices are convinced by impacts.

For example, think about a period that you see somebody gnawing his or her nails. In essence, you keep on watching this individual for a decent timeframe. You may logically review that, at one time you pursued the trail of this individual, therefore mirroring his or her conduct. By building up a higher plane of cognizance and mindfulness in any case, you can get yourself at the front position of time, rather than following the way of somebody that is guiding you wrong. Perceptions and affirmatives can enable you to build up that higher plane of cognizance and mindfulness. You receive rewards since while you are building up your aptitudes, you will likewise assemble enthusiastic competency. This procedure of advancement is exceptionally fundamental, given that feelings for quite a long time have gotten numerous individuals in a difficult situation. Some of you may think it is ridiculous to concentrate on something that you don't have. You may feel that representation is a psychological issue, though the individual thinks that it's hard to remain associated with the real world. The truth of the matter is we as a whole have perceptions, and we can utilize these mental pictures in the brain to move us through self-improvement.

From start to finish, we as a whole should progress in the self-advancement forms. Self-development empowers us to expand on our natural aptitudes and capacities. We have numerous advancement qualities to consider while traveling through these stages.

Start Your Day with Physical Activities

Physical movement invigorates the arrival of hormones to support your state of mind, kick off your vitality, battle pressure, and that's just the beginning. Being dynamic toward the beginning of the day may be exceptionally gainful. Research demonstrates that introduction to early morning light can enable you to feel progressively alert during the day, just as improve the nature of your rest around evening time.

These things can signify expanded profitability at work. Underneath, I've collected a portion of the science-supported ways that morning activity can help your business achievement. There are likewise some essential hints for pressing in new exercises.

Exercise and profitability

Exercise has a multi-pronged impact with regards to upgrading your presentation at work. It supports stamina and battles weariness. However, it likewise advances a quiet, engaged perspective that can enable you to do your best work - among its numerous advantages:

Discipline gives you more vitality. You may imagine that working out would further drain your vitality holds. Be that as it may, only 20 minutes of low-to-direct power work out (like strolling) performed three times each week can expand vitality levels by 20 percent and diminishing exhaustion by 65 percent, as indicated by a University of Georgia consider. The standard movement builds the course and reinforces your heart muscle, giving you more continuance to control through your bustling day.

Lift your mind-set. If you had an awful day, you realize how hard it very well may be to do your best work. Exercise invigorates the arrival of endorphins - synthetics that limit uneasiness and advance sentiments of remuneration and prosperity. You'll begin to feel these impacts inside only five minutes of beginning your exercise, American Psychological Association specialists.

Goes about as pressure the board apparatus. Exercise doesn't merely build feel-great endorphins. It additionally brings down degrees of stress hormones like cortisol and adrenaline, helping you feel more settled and increasingly loose. Furthermore, after some time, those advantages could indeed include: One creature concentrate found that regular exercise redesigns portions of the cerebrum, making it less receptive to push.

Hones your perception. Neuroscientists have long realized that physical action battles aggravation in mind and animates the development of new neurons. That could be the reason portions of the mind identified with intuition and memory are more significant in individuals who usually exercise contrasted with the individuals who don't, state Harvard Health specialists.

Why morning exercises are ideal

Exercise can build your profitability in a few various ways. Also, for various reasons, morning exercises might be much progressively powerful.

You'll skirt fewer exercises. Exercise's beneficial outcomes are combined - you have to work out reliably to keep up the advantages. It's normal for tasks, gatherings and off the cuff charitable solicitations to control evening or night exercise plans off base. However, when you practice in the first part of the day, there are fewer diversions to avoid.

You'll feel increasingly conscious. Exercise can't supplant a decent night's rest. In any case, the flow and endorphin support that accompany an exercise can enable you to get moving in the first part of the day. That is particularly valid if you take your action outside since presentation to morning light advances alertness and lifts psychological execution, as indicated by a Swiss report.

You'll have a simpler time dozing during the evening. Regular exercisers will, in general, rest better contrasted with the inactive individuals. Furthermore, discoveries recommend that moving in the first part of the day could be particularly valuable: People who exercise at 7 a.m. invest 75 percent more energy in the most profound phases of rest than the individuals who exercise toward the evening or night, as indicated by a Journal of Strength and Conditioning Research contemplate.

Chapter 8 Military Discipline and Self-discipline

Soldiers were taught to be disciplined and obedient. They had to follow authority, commands, and rules without question. If they question the authority, then it becomes a problem. To be considered well-disciplined, the team has to follow orders whether they like it or not, and no matter how unpleasant and dangerous the task at hand is.

Total compliance is required to achieve efficiency within the organization. Disorganization and disobedience in the team is dangerous and can put the lives of the other group members at risk. The survival of the military groups and special forces units depend a lot on the obedience of the team to a centralized command and the self-discipline of each and every member.

Military self-discipline is achieved when the soldier starts to see himself as an integral instrument to achieve the organization's mission. This internalization involves acceptance of regulation and obedience to a higher authority. Soldiers who are self-disciplined know how to control themselves and always make decisions based on how it will affect the entire organization. They also do not need to constant external supervision because they know how to keep themselves in line.

When a soldier has self-discipline, obedience comes from within and not from coercion or other form of external force. Those soldiers who exhibit strong willpower and self-discipline are viewed by their superior as reliable. The higher-ups know that these soldiers can perform their duty correctly and willingly, without the need to use force or coercion. These highly disciplined soldiers are the ones who move up to become members of the highly elite special forces or special operations units.

Special Forces Training

Of course, the different units of the elite Special Forces have different kinds of training but they are more or less the same. They are all physically, mentally, and emotionally demanding, exhausting, and intensive. Their training is a lot more difficult than the training of regular soldiers. This is because they will be assigned to work in high-risk and high-profile operations that affect not only their own country but the whole world.

The Special Forces training is the toughest training and testing platform in the Military. It is a year-long process that is designed to break even the toughest soldiers. In fact, it is so difficult to pass that only 15% of the candidates successfully finish the entire process.

Once you enter the training, you only have three options—to quit, get injured, or outlast—and of course the third option is the only option if you want to become a member of the Special Forces group. You are probably wondering how can an individual survive such training if it is designed to break even the toughest person.

Keep in mind that the human body is a wonderful machine and can adapt in almost all kinds of situation—heat, cold, pain, and stress. Someone who is tough means that his body and also his mind and emotions are highly adaptable and does not easily give up because he knows that it is possible to successfully complete the training. More often than not, it is mind over matter.

The training also puts a lot of emphasis on mental strength aside from physical strength. If the body is strong enough to withstand pain and discomfort, it becomes easy to develop mental strength.

- The right mindset

Members of these Special Forces Units are highly self-disciplined because they have the right mindset. Self-discipline has more to do with mental toughness than physical toughness, although mental toughness becomes easier to achieve if the body is also strong.

If you want to be successful in life, you have to stick it out until the end even when things become too hard to handle. This is something that the Special Forces have—when the going gets tough, they still continue doing their mission, something that the rest of the society should learn.

The world you live in today is filled with softies who get offended at the smallest things and if you develop mental toughness like the Special Forces, then you have an advantage over all these people. You are setting yourself up for success when you have the mindset to stick it out while the rest is giving up.

- Physical training

The Special Forces Units have to undergo intensive physical training, as you already know by now. The kind of physical training that they do require a lot more than being strong and healthy. To be able to successfully do all the physical tests, you have to have commitment and self-discipline. Principles included in the training are work capacity, calisthenics or gymnastics, resistance training, and endurance, to name a few.

This kind of training gives Special Forces soldiers a strong and athletic body that is well-rounded and can perform well in any kind of weather and environment and even in extremely stressful situations.

You do not necessarily need to follow the difficult training of the Spartans and the Special Forces Units and you do not need to train at that level because you are just an ordinary person who wants to improve your life by obtaining self-discipline. However, the information and facts shared in this chapter will at least give you an idea how the Spartans and Special Forces train that greatly improves their self-discipline, and you can use what you have learned to greatly improve your self-discipline. At least you know one thing now—being successful takes a lot of hard work and effort on your part. It is not a walk in the park.

The Science and Psychology of Self-Discipline

One of the most famous psychological tests is the marshmallow test, which you are probably very familiar with. It is a part of a series of studies on willpower and delayed gratification. The studies were conducted by a Stanford professor Walter Mischel in the 60s and 70s. Even back then, experts were very much interested in understanding willpower. And up to know, psychologists and scientist still conduct studies about it because it unlocks to key to a successful life.

Willpower gives us self-discipline. It is what prevents us from spending all our money buying things that we like and instead putting them in a savings account for the future. It is what makes us go to work and finish our job before the deadline or study for an exam even when all we want to do is watch TV or sleep. It is what pushes us to eat healthy and spend an hour at the gym exercising. It is what makes us say no to temptations,

temptations that will give us instant gratification but will sabotage our future.

No wonder scientists and psychologist continue to study willpower and self-discipline. It is what makes a person successful. They want to understand what makes a person more disciplined than the next person, and in what situation and what is the reasoning behind it. What exactly is going on in the brain, chemically speaking, when a person summons up his willpower to force himself to do things he really does not want to do to get his reward later on, and also when a person just gives up and says, to hell with it? These have been a topic of discussion and research for decades.

Components of achieving goals

Although willpower and self-discipline are considered the key to a successful life, other things also play important roles in achieving goals and objectives. The first thing that you need to do is to know your motivation and set a clear goal. The Spartans, for instance, were motivated to undergo the training because they want to become citizens and also to be someone worthy in the eyes of their people.

The Special Forces are motivated because they know that they are going to be a part of an elite team that plays an important role in world issues and conflicts. Your motivation can be something as simple as wanting to provide a good life for your family or wanting to look and feel good.

The second component is monitoring your behavior towards that goal. You have to want it badly enough to be able to endure hardships and challenges that you might encounter in trying to achieve your goal. Your behavior should not change while in the process of achieving your goal. Otherwise, you will lose the reason why you are doing all of those things in the first place.

And finally, the third component of achieving goals is willpower that leads to self-discipline. You cannot achieve your goal without the willpower to overcome temptations. Whether it is saying no to another chocolate bar, not watching random YouTube videos, or stopping yourself from buying something just because it is on sale, willpower plays an important role in all this.

The energy model of self-control

This is one of the popular theories about willpower and self-discipline, that states that the brain works like a muscle. It has a supply of strength or energy that is limited and can be used up through exertion. This is why we have lapses when it comes to willpower. We are not self-disciplined at all times because our mental energy for self-control is depleted, also called ego depletion.

If you have used up your mental energy by practicing willpower and self-control to do one particular task, then it might be difficult to be as disciplined as before with subsequent challenges. This is the reason why we are more prone to give in to instant gratifications, such as going on a shopping spree or eating sweets, when we are feeling stressed. It suffers from fatigue after usage but just like an ordinary muscle, it can also be strengthened through exercise, meaning you have to continue using it again and again to make your willpower stronger. The effect of fatigue is instant while the effect of strengthening the muscle is delayed.

There was an experiment conducted to show that willpower is a limited resource. Two groups of individuals were placed in the same room, one group was given a bowl of cookies that were freshly baked and smelled really good, and the other group was given a bowl of radishes. First group was told to eat the cookies and the second group was told to eat the radishes.

After some time, the participants were given a puzzle to solve. And not surprisingly, those who ate cookies kept working on the puzzle for 20 minutes while those who ate the radishes only lasted a measly 8 minutes. The explanation behind this is that the participants who ate the radishes already used their brain energy or willpower to resist eating the delicious-smelling cookies. They did not have any more energy reserves to continue solving the puzzle.

But aside from exerting willpower again and again, the brain also suffers more from the so-called ego depletion when they are practicing self-discipline to please others and not to achieve personal goals and desires. This is why it is best to set clear goals that will benefit yourself and not to impress others.

According to the proponents of this theory, mental energy can be refueled by simply providing your brain with sugar or other simple carbohydrates. This model has been tremendously influential in a lot of succeeding studies about willpower and self-discipline.

But what actually gets depleted when a person no longer has the energy to control himself? Willpower is a term used to describe psychological processes that is happening in the brain but what exactly is the scientific process? Glucose plays an important role in this theory. It acts as a fuel that helps the brain perform mental activities efficiently. Anything that your body does is fueled by glucose—muscular exertion and function of the immune system. Neurotransmitters are also composed of glucose. Glucose comes from sugar and also other nutritious foods. It is either used right away or stored as energy reserves for later use.

However, it cannot be said that it is the be-all and end-all explanation. There is more to self-discipline than refueling the brain with sugar.

Defining self-discipline

Self-discipline can be used interchangeably with these terms: willpower, drive, determination, self-control, and resolve. But what exactly is self-discipline? It is a person's ability to not give in to impulses, behaviors, and emotions that will give instant rewards in order to achieve long-term goals.

This is what separates humans from animals, which has scientific basis because the whole process of willpower and self-discipline happens in the pre-frontal cortex of the brain, which is a lot bigger in humans than in animals, particularly other mammals with the same kind of brain structure. Some scientists even go as far as claiming that self-discipline is what makes humans human. This allows humans to plan and analyze alternate course of actions instead of doing whatever they feel like doing that can only lead to regret. It is the ability to wait for a bigger reward by forgoing small and easy rewards.

It is also the capacity to remove any unwanted feeling, thought, or impulse especially when you are having a difficult time. The Spartans and Special Forces probably have thought about quitting or giving up during the difficult training but they have the mental strength not to give up because they focus their sight on their goals.

There are three different aspects of willpower, or self-discipline: the ability to resist impulses and temptations or the "I won't" power, the ability to do things that have to be done or the "I will" power, and the awareness of your personal desires and goals or the "I want" power. You have to use all these three not only to achieve your goals but also to steer clear of trouble.

Self-discipline is a form of effortful and conscious regulation of one's self by one's self. It is all about fighting temptations, resisting impulses, and using different kinds of techniques to be in control. No wonder it is a tiring activity, because your enemy is your own self.

Delaying gratification

The popular marshmallow experiment stated previously is a prime example of delayed gratification. Willpower is basically that, the ability of an individual to delay gratification. The lead researcher gave a more detailed explanation using the hot and cool systems.

The cool system is a thinking system responsible for analyzing feelings, actions, and sensations. It is a reflective system that reminds you why you should not eat that marshmallow right away.

Then there is the hot system, which is emotional and impulsive, and reacts quickly to external stimuli and triggers, such as eating the marshmallow right away because you know how fluffy and sweet it would taste and feel in your mouth. Just think of it this way, the cool system is the angel and the hot system is the devil.

When the hot system overrides the cool system in your brain, meaning your willpower fails, you give in to temptations and impulses because it makes you feel good at that instant. According to these studies, some people are more sensitive to impulses and emotional triggers, which is why they are more likely to give in to temptations.

Why Self-discipline is important

You already know by now that self-discipline is an important factor to reach your goals. The Spartans and Special Forces soldiers will not reach that level of success in achieving their goals if they do not practice self-discipline. Sure, it is just one piece of the puzzle but it is definitely an important piece. It is an essential tool if you want to be successful in life.

For instance, self-discipline played a bigger role when it comes to academic success than IQ. You may be smart and intelligent, but if you do not have the self-discipline to attend classes, submit projects on time, or to study for an exam, you will still get lower grades.

If you are a disciplined and conscientious student who studies every night instead of chatting with friends and watching videos, wakes up early every day and attends classes on time, and finishes projects and submits them before the deadline, you will surely get a higher grade.

Education or attending school is not just about learning new things and acquiring knowledge. It is also about developing your self-discipline to do things that you really do not want to do but you are expected to do to become successful in life.

And when you go out to the real world, your willpower and self-discipline is tested on a daily basis. You might be tempted to stay in bed and call in sick because you do not feel like working. But you still get up and you force yourself to go to work because you need to earn money.

You might be tempted to use your credit card to buy that expensive designer bag that you really, really want. But you don't because you know your salary can't afford it and you don't really need a bag that costs thousands of dollars. Everyday you are faced with such temptations and impulses and every day you fight them. You might get tired, sure, but it is something that you really have to do if you want to achieve your long-term goals, such as saving up for the future.

Moreover, most of the problems that people face in today's world are related to self-discipline or self-control. These include addiction, alcoholism, large debt, unwanted pregnancy, domestic violence, crimes, overeating, sexually transmitted disease, lack of savings, educational failure, underperformance at work, and so on and so forth. The list continues and it's all because people do not have the willpower or self-discipline. This only shows that self-discipline is powerful and should be utilized in order to become a successful individual. Making the decision to improve your self-discipline is the first step towards success.

This also helps us interact better with other people in the society. Just imagine if you do not practice self-discipline. You will just say whatever is on your mind or do whatever you feel like doing without thinking about consequences of your actions. Rules and regulations in a society go hand in hand with discipline. Without these rules and regulations in place, the world will be a dangerous and scary place to live in. And we follow these rules because we have self-discipline.

Chapter 9 Your Friendship With Pain

Pain will be something you will have to confront. Most humans run when they are confronted by pain. Whenever you take positive actions like going to the gym, quit smoking, writing that report, eating healthy or getting up early, you might feel pain. You will feel discomfort. Your first thought will be to stop. This is where most people end their effort with Self-Discipline.

They start feeling discomfort and they give up. They feel pain the first time and immediately stop. They want to go back to comfort now. Instant gratification is what they want. They can't take the pain a bit longer to get the results they want. So, they give up and run to comfort.

These shadows in our minds are scary for most humans. When they go into these territories in their minds for the first time, they resist it, they turn around and run.

What you need to do is turn around and confront the pain. Make friends with it. When you start feeling discomfort smile at it and own it. Tell yourself that its fine to feel pain or discomfort. Once you feel the pain realize that this is your signal that you are doing the right thing. Walk through the darkness. Start loving these experiences because you know they are making you stronger.

People Don't Like Change

The obvious thing about self-discipline is that you need to change. But there is another thing that plagues humans. This is the fact that Humans hate change.

Most people will never change. Especially in today's comfortable environment where people get anything they want with the press of a button. They get seduced by modern comfort. So, they delay change and improvement.

That is why things like new year's resolutions never work. People are too comfortable and they want the instant gratification. So, most people never change. Life goes on and before you know it all kinds of chaos has broken out.

For example, a person starts to get overweight and thinks about losing some weight by starting a new workout plan. So, the person tells himself he will start in 3 weeks when the new year starts. So, the new year starts, and nothing happens. He thought about change for a few minutes but then got seduced by comfort and that doughnut on the table. He didn't listen to his friend who told him to be disciplined and start exercising and eating healthy.

So, what happens? Biology strikes hard and ruthlessly. A year later he becomes seriously ill and the doctor says he is a diabetic. Something he could have prevented if he had self-discipline and took control of his life.

So yes, biology waits for nobody. But in today's environment, there is another enemy that is allowed to seduce and comfort the masses of people out there. This enemy is feelings. The modern world is addicted to feelings.

They have given feelings absolute priority over everything else. If someone feels sad, angry, depressed and bad then the world has to stop and comfort that person. The world has been seduced by this addiction to feelings.

They have traded truth for comfort. They won't point out problems they will hide behind feelings. When a person can't walk up the stairs, they will not say you are fat. They will say, "He is just a little tired".

When a person failed his test, they won't say "You are lazy", they will say "He had a bad day".

When someone is late, they won't point out the bad manners they will just say "That's ok".

We hide from the truth so we can feel comfy and coddled. In most developed countries like the US, Canada, and Europe people live in coddled spoilt societies. The results of this are that society as a whole is becoming weaker and weaker. Today's society gives each other hugs for everything. But unfortunately, what many people need is slap in the face to wake up from the trance they are in.

This leads to people really struggling on an individual level to change when they have to. This also makes people give up very easily when they decide they want to change. They are mentally weak.

We mentioned the importance of accepting pain earlier in this chapter. The problem is that in today's world pain is avoided at all costs. The brutal reality of biology is that the clock is ticking and your time is running out. Every second you allow yourself to get seduced by emotion, warm hugs, participation trophies and modern comforts you are getting deeper into trouble.

Here is another newsflash. If you don't make the changes necessary to live your best life you will probably live a life of depression, unhappiness, and stress. This is just how biology rips comfort to pieces. Again, biology has no feelings whatsoever and if you don't get on the same playing field by adapting Self-Discipline you will lose. And lose badly.

Let me use an analogy to explain how it goes in life for most people. Let's imagine every person on this planet is on a ship on the ocean. This ship represents your life. This ship is made up of your life story. This ship includes everything. The way you live, what you eat, your lifestyle and self-discipline or the lack of self-discipline.

Now let's imagine everyone wants to go North because North is where success is. The problem is that most people that have no Self- Discipline in their lives think they are going North but they are actually heading South. South is where the rocks are. The rocks mean danger and death. Most people end up on the rocks.

So, what happens when people hit the rocks? They freak out and act surprised. They don't know what happened. They don't understand how everything around them turned into chaos. Then they start remembering the new year's resolutions they didn't follow through on. They remember the time spent partying when they should have been studying. They remember all those doughnuts and ice cream they ate when should have been eating healthy. But now it's too late.

Don't be one of those people who is going in the wrong direction. You need to realize the seriousness of the situation and make the changes necessary so you can go North.

What To Do If You Are On The Rocks Now?

If you are on the rocks now then I have some good news and some bad news. The good news is that you can still make it north. The bad news is you will have to not only accept pain as a friend, but you will also have to make it your brother. You will need to look for the pain. You will need to embrace pain so that you become so strong that the natural momentum of your efforts pushes you north.

The Bottom Line Of Self Discipline

You need to learn to do things you hate. The world we live in today tells us to just be comfortable and that we should avoid things we don't like. This is the biggest reason why so many people don't get what they want in life. To get what you want you to need to accept the following point: You have to start doing things you don't like doing. In fact, you need to become excellent at those things that you don't like doing.

A lot of people walk around saying that "I just want to follow my heart or my passion". Listen, that whole idea was built in a dream world. In reality, even the people that do things they love for a living sometimes have to do things they hate.

Talk to the most successful people on the planet and they will tell you the same thing. Sure, I agree, find the thing you love, but to get there you might have to walk through a lot of crap. And guess what? Once you achieve the thing you want you still need to do some things you hate. This is the real world.

A lot of people quit their jobs and start their own businesses and then get a rude awakening. They thought now that they work for themselves, they only get to do things they love. Unfortunately, the world of business doesn't work that way. Anything of value on this planet takes discipline and hard work to turn into reality.

This way of thinking is unfortunately widespread in the world we live in. It's especially prevalent in the online world of business and social media. The internet has created a massive opportunity for many people to create a living online and this has created the false idea of overnight success.

The whole modern entertainment industry including social media and others has created the false reality of overnight success. People buy into this idea of becoming rich and famous overnight. They see the post on social media showing someone posing in a car full of cash. The guy in the car says he became rich in a month and you can do the same. People buy into this rubbish.

Unfortunately, we now have a culture of entitlement. People want all their dreams to come true right now. They don't want to hear about things like hard work, perseverance. patience and self-discipline. They want the magic pill, the quick fix so that they can get that warm fussy feeling inside. The last thing they want is to do things they hate to get what they want. All they want is the big check and the pictures on social media.

You see it everywhere. In business, people start online and the first thing they ask is how they can outsource most of the work. I have nothing against delegating and outsourcing. However, that should not be your first priority. In fact, you need to do the hard work yourself first to get a better understanding of how your business works and what your employees go through. You need to do the hard work first before you earn the right to start playing the big boss man.

In fitness, people see their favorite movie star on TV and they think I want to look like that guy. The first thing they start looking for is some kind of supplement or protein powder that will build them that physique. They don't start with a workout and start doing the hard work necessary to get that body. In my own life, I hate running but I still do it because it gets me where

I want to go in terms of my fitness and health goals. The upside of running totally outweighs the downside of my feelings towards running.

With dating and relationships, it's the same. A guy sees a beautiful woman somewhere and he asks his coworker to go ask the girl for her phone number. He doesn't have the courage to get into the "uncomfortable" situation and go talk to the girl. He wants all the upside with no downside.

Self-Discipline will teach you how to shut out all these voices in your head trying to stop you from success. Your discipline will keep you in check when you don't want to do the hard work necessary to get to where you want to go. It's now up to you to do the hard work to build a culture of Self Discipline in your life.

Chapter 10 Pareto Principle

Do you want to know the secret to accomplishing great goals?

The answer may surprise you. In fact, what I'm about to suggest will maybe strike a chord with you and make you think I am crazy.

I assure you I am not.

What I'm going to recommend, is for you to do less.

That's correct less.

In order to maximize your best efforts, you need to concentrate them and by concentrating them on better outcomes you accomplish what you set out to accomplish.

You will find that it is better for your health, for your stress levels, for your relationships with loved ones, and for everything else that matters to you.

What I am talking about was identified by Vifredo Pareto, who made the distinction that 80% of Italy's land was owned by 20% of the population.

He began looking at other countries and found this to be true in every instance that he looked. It was the same distribution pattern in effect.

The Pareto principle looked at processes in just about every field from engineering to sociology, economy, politics, anything you could basically think of the vast majority of time, the competition for resources was dominated by 20% in some cases it may even more pronounced.

So, what does this mean to you? How can you apply this to your life to make things better to move ahead at an accelerated pace and identify the tasks and functions you do that are the most important to your job? For example, if your job is that of an accountant, you will be better served working on client work that gives you income other tasks such as answering the phone, responding to emails, and all of the other functions that happen in an office which would probably be better utilized by hiring someone to come in and perform those duties for you so you can spend your attention and resources on the things that matter to your bottom line.

This also works in sports. In the sport of Brazilian jujitsu there are literally thousands of moves that can be performed to subdue an opponent. However, there is an almost disparaging number of times in high level tournaments that one very basic move that a new practitioner will learn within several months of beginning training can use at even the highest levels. For example, if in a match, the opponent winds up on the back of the other opponent and chokes the person or submits him or her. They have found that particular move is utilized and successful in more than 60 to 70% of matches at the highest level. In other words, the 80/20 rule works here as well. It shows that just a handful of moves in each position will yield nearly all of the results versus the other moves combined.

Somewhere else this can be looked at is in the field of politics. Politics such as in the American system, the party of the Republicans and the Democrats dominates the political scene.

There are hundreds of other private parties such as Libertarians, the Green party, the Communist Party, the socialist party, and on and on and on but we never hear anything about them. They never make a strong run for party dominance, except maybe at the local level. At the national level, it will always be between the two major parties and everyone else is a very distant second. By taking this principle and applying it to your work. I believe it is easy to see just how important this principle is going forward. Do not focus on the busywork in front of you and on the long to do list you have written in your daytime or on your calendar program on your phone. Instead, focus only on the tasks they give you the most bang for your buck. You will know what they are and they are specific to you but if you follow this as I've laid out.

I believe you will make significant progress and it makes self-discipline that much easier because now you are only focusing in on a few different habits to give yourself. You are not focusing on the entire picture of productivity and self-discipline, instead what you are focusing on are just a couple of different things that will get you ahead in the fastest amount of time possible.

You can apply to developing self-discipline as well. Instead of making a huge list of foods you can't eat, instead focus on just a few foods that you know are healthful and tasty. You do not have to think about the myriad choices that abound and simply focus on the few that give you the most benefit. Or, you can use a simple rule that says you will always have a protein source in each meal. This simplifies things.

How about batching your email and only checking it once or twice a day? You will save time and energy as well as be more productive by cutting your email response time down to 20% of your time instead of the 80% you may be spending now.

Try making goals that cut across different disciplines of your life. Becoming a better listener can help you become a better spouse, parent, manager, business owner. Getting to be a better budgeter can help you at home and at your job.

So, by adopting a few key habits you can have profound impact in many different areas of your life instead of adopting a bunch of new habits.

Chapter 11 Look for Micro Improvements

1% Improvement. It may not seem like much, but the fact of the matter is we are either improving or declining a little each and every day.

If you look at as an X and Y axis aligned going straight up and going straight across. If you put your life right in the middle going parallel to the X axis. You can see that there will be either gradual trend upwards or gradual trends downwards.

This can be discouraging, if you look at it wrong.

You may think 'I don't have control over that, that is just the way my life is going.'

Or it can be sobering if you truly see how the little things you do each day will add up no matter what. They can be good or bad, they do not judge.

The process is called aggregate gains. It is the compound effect of either a good or a bad habit.

Let's look at several examples. If you never miss a workout then over time, the aggregate gain will be solid fitness.

Let's say your nutrition is something you struggle with and continue to make poor food choices day in and day out, you will find yourself overweight and with preventable diseases such as heart disease and diabetes.

Small wins and slow gains, according to James Clear are the goal. The system is where it is at and you need to master your habits. Do not aim for huge changes all at once.

Having huge goals is wonderful but it is also intimidating and can actually bring down your enthusiasm. Eventually it will lead to inaction and over analysis and you will develop difficulty making progress. The little things will stress you and make you uncomfortable and zap your energy.

Set small goals, create a system for accomplishing that small goal and experience the win.

Make the process the goal.

What you do not want to do is this. Don't think about the big picture all the time, simply use that as a rudder towards where you were going.

Pretend you are swimming in a lake and headed toward an island in the middle of a lake. Will you get impatient if you are not at the lake within a certain amount of time? Will you tell yourself that you should have been there already? Of course not, you will get there when you get there. However, if you look up occasionally to see if you're on track and not headed in the wrong direction that is okay. The goal is simply something you are aiming for; the swimming is the key. Concentrating on smooth strokes, conserving your energy etc are the immediate goals that will get you to the island. Concentrating on anything else and you can drown.

You just do not want to become consumed with the idea of not accomplishing your goal. You are moving toward your goal and are making progress, even if it does not feel like it because the water is deep and cold.

James Clear also says to focus on the daily process and enjoy the present moment and succeed.

It is called the kaizen approach, which is Japanese for continuous improvement.

It emphasizes making small improvements each day. Think of the smallest step you can take every day to achieve that goal. It can be as simple as sending an email to a potential client, even if it is not hundred percent perfect. Or making a phone call to someone that you haven't spoken to in a long time and you need to mend that fence.

Poor nutrition? Try adding a protein source to each meal to counteract the other less desirable carbohydrates present.

So even if you aren't ready to completely alter your diet at least you're getting something a little more nutritionally sound to begin with. While you're at it, try to cut down on the empty calories. It leaves room for more healthy options.

Take the stairs for one flight of your journey to the office and then take the elevator for the rest, if your condition doesn't allow you to take the entire stairs to your office.

Meditate for one minute a day to start. You're more than likely to stay with that if you do this, increase it as needed.

Let's put some things in perspective. If you were to improve one thing 1% each day. Where would you end up? Laura Stack lays it out nicely. She says if you can improve 1% each day you would roughly double your ability every 70 days.

Think about the possibilities here. It is mind boggling. Just doing something 1% better each day. You will be a new person in a little over two months in that particular area.

For instance, let's say you want to listen to your spouse better just 1%. Imagine that if you did this your relationship with him or her would get better and better instead of possibly drifting apart with nothing to talk about.

Too often we try to do things when it's too late. We are already in over our head and we get overwhelmed.

With this 1% improvement mantra. We can take on huge projects and not be overwhelmed by them.

Just sit back right now and think about one thing you want to get better at.

Got it?

Now think about the smallest incremental step you can take to accomplish. It gives you the best chance of becoming the disciplined person you want to be. The person who does what they say they are going to do, no matter what. Say for instance you want to become more punctual begin getting ready five minutes earlier than you would normally begin getting ready.

Will you still be late? Maybe, but maybe not as late and as time goes on, you'll begin to see that you are becoming more and more punctual. This is the goal, it's not all at once. The change doesn't happen instantaneously. It happens gradually and in time. All of a sudden, you begin seeing yourself as a punctual person if not early to appointments. Devin from Project No Limits on YouTube wrote or says success is not overnight. It is a daily commitment. Think about old apprenticeships. They would work daily until they became proficient and eventually would become the master of their trade. For example, blacksmiths.

Improving your life is as easy as 1%. The first step is to look for at every opportunity is a way to improve. Perhaps you get mad when someone says something to you that triggers you, maybe now you decide I'm going to count to 10 before I respond. What will this do? It gives you a second to think now to not react like you had and all of a sudden, you're reacting to things 1% better than you did. Or let's say you can take a little thing such as eye contact. Say you want to hold eye contact better with people and noticed a change in the conversations that you have with those people. Are they improving? I'm sure they are and it may not even be noticeable, but they are.

Maybe improve your posture. Stand up a little straighter and it will seem like you are better overnight from doing that? Of course not, but what it does is gives you the ability to stand up straighter and with that posture improvement you feel better.

Another thing you can do read five pages a day, you'll learn something new each and every day and you will become more interesting to other people around you. You will also become smarter and learn more things and be more disciplined and you'll finish more books.

Do this for a year when you think happens?

Do you get 365% better if you did 1% improvement each day for a year? The answer will surprise you, and that is no, you will not get 365% better. What you will get is a thousand to 2000% better because the effects compound each other.

They build upon each other. It's like compound interest in your finances.

How do you get started? Look at small areas. Organize something in your life that is bugging you. Maybe there's a bookshelf or your desk that is messy. Clean it and all of a sudden you are feeling more like the person that cleans their workspace and works in a clean, organized environment. Perhaps now you are known as the person who is organized and maybe you weren't before.

Do it day in and day out.

Write down the one thing you want to start with 1% improvement on a Post-it note commit to doing it for three days. Do this and see where you're at in a year's time. If you stick with it. I can almost guarantee you your life will change for the better and dramatically.

Chapter 12 Daily Habits That Can Increase Your Level of Self-Discipline

Have an Attitude of Gratitude

Gratitude comes with a whole lot of benefits, from improving the state of your mental health to enhancing your emotional wellbeing. Most importantly, gratitude helps you detach from your state of lack and scarcity. Thinking about the things you desire will make it hard for you to attain the level of self-discipline you need to actually achieve your goals.

FORGIVE

When it comes to forgiveness, you must learn to forgive both yourself and others to enable you to get ahead in life. Learning to forgive yourself when you err and others when they hurt you is an act of discipline that helps build up your energy for success. Whenever people hurt you, just forgive them and empty your mind of a load of hate and malice. Forgiving people who hurt you helps you release all negative energy that makes you lose your self-discipline. You must get rid of that negative energy, because holding it will make you feel tired, discouraged, and angry all the time. Plus, it subtracts from your capability of thinking.

MEDITATE

Engaging in meditations helps put your mind at ease. It creates a type of spiritual atmosphere around you to help you grow and become a better you. Meditation sets the stage for you to attain a higher state of self-discipline by clearing the palette of your mind and putting you in the right mood to face the challenges of the day.

Set Active Goals for Each Day

Active goals are active because they can be seen. You make your goals active by putting them down on paper and placing them where they can be seen. Active goals help you build and increase your level of self-discipline, because they give your life daily direction. This is when I talk about daily activities. There's no need to have an extreme objective or dream to set active goals; in fact, there are activities, such as washing the clothes, reading books, cooking, sleeping 8 hours a day, etc., that you will need to do every day. You can start with those home activities to increase your self-discipline.

Eat Right

When you eat the right foods, you help your body store more energy. When your diet is mostly composed of fats, carbohydrates, and proteins, your body dissipates lots of energy processing such foods. When you eat more fruits and veggies, which require less energy to be processed, you will experience an energy boost that will help you pursue your goals with an adequate level of self-discipline. Also, eating at the same time every day will help you to have a healthy life when it comes to ingesting the right nutrients. This way you will avoid having diseases or stomach problems, such as gastritis. Having these health problems will only take part of your time to recover, and you will have to postpone your goals. It is preferable to prevent than to cure.

Get Enough Sleep

There is a direct link between sleep and self-discipline. Whether you give your body enough rest by getting adequate sleep or not goes a long way to determine your ability to stay focused on your goal to achieve self-discipline, and your general wellbeing. Make sure you get 6-8 hours of sleep, no matter how busy you are.

Exercise Daily

Incorporating physical exercises into your daily routines helps you get rid of bad habits and adopt positive habits. If you really want to learn to discipline yourself, make certain physical exercises part of your morning routine. Most people give the excuse that they are too busy or have a lot of worries to get involved in physical exercises. Where such people get it wrong is that they forget they can improve their entire lives through physical exercise.

Stay Organized

Don't just wake up and start working on your goals for the day. Make sure you have your goals and daily tasks arranged in an orderly manner. Arranging your goals in an orderly manner helps you stay organized which is a good sign of self-discipline. Being organized goes beyond having a list of things to do, taking into account priorities. It also involves organizing all areas of your life such as your work table, your drawer, your kitchen cabinets, your wardrobe, your garage, your bedroom, and all other such spaces in your life.

READ

The body is not everything and health does not imply only work out the body. You also have to work out your mind and improve your knowledge and intelligence. There's no better way to do this than reading a book. It is considered one of the best habits a person may have and will definitely guide you to accomplishing your goals. Reading opens the mind to new worlds and offers new life perspectives. I always recommend reading books often. You will learn from it, and you will find different ways to perform your daily activities. You can find encouragement in this, improve your reading and writing skills, and feel more confident in any aspect of your life, due to the acquired knowledge.

Chapter 13 How Zen Philosophy Can Help You Achieve Your Goals

Wouldn't it be wonderful to know that whatever life throws at you, you'll be able to process it and move on? Wouldn't it be great to live free from that underlying anxiety you feel whenever change looms large on the horizon? What about losing your fear of never having done quite enough with your life, and even feeling comfortable with the inevitability of death? You're about to learn the basics of an ancient philosophy that has been enriching Eastern lives for thousands of years. In this chapter we're going to look at Buddhist philosophy, with a concentration on Zen. You'll learn how it can help you develop a greater level of self-discipline and move you closer to achieving your goals. Over the past couple of decades, researchers in psychology and self-development fields have noticed that Zen practitioners often enjoy good psychological health. Researchers at Penn State University have spent over a decade looking at the effects of practices associated with Zen, including meditation. It turns out that weaving Buddhist principles into your everyday life can lower stress, induce feelings of calm and help you make better decisions.

Zen Buddhists can teach us a lot about delaying gratification, overcoming fear and accomplishing our goals. This lays a powerful foundation for self-discipline. Zen is not in itself a religion. It's best thought of as a kind of experience, a way of life based on the teachings of the Buddha. The closest Japanese term for Zen is "satori," which roughly translates to "first showing" or "flash of inspiration." To experience Zen is to live in the presence, and fully appreciate that everything is connected. This state is said to be extremely hard to put into words, but roughly speaking it entails a suspension of the self and ego.

To put Zen philosophy into context, it helps to know a little about the life of Buddha. Several thousand years ago, he began spreading the teachings and observations which had led to his enlightenment. In short, he taught two key ideas. His first idea was that suffering was very much a part of human life. His second was that for the most part, we bring it on ourselves. Having left his life of luxury to go out into the world and learn about the true nature of existence, he noted that the majority of people were bound in a state of misery. He eventually concluded that if we are to break free of the endless cycle of birth, suffering and rebirth, we have to stop allowing our minds to grasp onto the illusions and attachments that we tend to hold onto.

These attachments include our very sense of self. For example, when we are with someone else there is no "I" or "you," just two humans who have created the illusion of two separate egos using the power of their own minds. The aim of Buddhism, and of Zen in particular, is to strip away the incessant mind chatter and illusions we hold about the outside world and realize on a deep level that everything is interconnected. There is no "us" and "them," no "in here and "out there." Once we attain this level of insight, the concerns of society – such as acquiring social status and material possessions – will come to matter a whole lot less. Instead, we can focus on moral development and lead a much more balanced life. We'll also save ourselves much unnecessary suffering by letting go of the notion that external events can make us happy.

Buddhism encourages living life in the present moment. The past is merely a set of memories and set of interpretations. The future has yet to arrive, and obsessing or worrying about particular outcomes will only lead to pointless mental suffering.

This may sound a bit abstract and spiritual. A couple of examples from everyday life will help you better understand how it all fits together.

Take the issue of self-identity. Zen teaches us that holding on too tightly to a rigid idea about who you are and what this means is self-limiting and keeps you locked in the same destructive behavior patterns. When I started reading about Zen for the first time, I soon realized that I had long had a self-image as a high achiever. This sounds like a good problem to have, right? Well yes – in a sense. But if you have a similar self-image, you'll know that it comes at a cost to your mental health. When you are told from an early age that you're smart, grades and career success will become a major focus in your life as a child and then as an adult. This leaves you at risk of stress and burnout.

Worse still, the prospect of failure becomes scarier over time as you cling tighter and tighter to the idea that you are, and must remain, a high achiever. As if that wasn't enough, you fall into the trap of striving for qualifications that don't actually make you happy. Think about it. Have you become permanently happier with each new accolade or qualification? Probably not. It's more likely that you have felt increasingly anxious about being "found out" or revealed to be a fraud. By this point, if you experience failure then your self-image will unravel and your world will tip upside down. People hate the possibility that their lives might slide out of control (and I'm not immune to this either).

Incorporating Zen principles and the teachings of Buddha into your life will help you develop self-discipline and ultimately achieve your goals. Why? Firstly, you will accept that since suffering is inevitable, you should be prepared to work for whatever it is you want. Second, you will gain more control over your own mind. Rather than losing hours to pointless rumination and regrets, you'll be busy appreciating what's going on in the present. Third, you will feel less constrained by fear. After all, fear is just an inevitable result of thinking about all the potential ways in which things could go wrong. If you don't allow your mind to dwell on all the negative possibilities, fear will no longer hold you back. Your thought processes will be sharper and you will be calmer, because you will no longer be fighting against a flood of negative thoughts.

Now let's go back to the issue of goals. You'd be forgiven for thinking that if **Buddhism** encourages you to dissolve the boundaries between your ego and the world around you whilst refusing to dwell on the future, there's little room left for setting and working towards goals. Yet this isn't the case. The Buddha himself outlined a spiritual framework known as The Eightfold Path, which includes guidelines such as "right speech," "right view," and "right action." Not only are these guidelines distinctly proactive in themselves – you can't get much more proactive than "right action"– but they are definitely goals. Therefore, there is no contradiction between adding the central ideas of Zen into your life whilst looking to improve it at the same time.

Mastering Self-Discipline The Shaolin Way

Now that you understand the key ideas behind Zen and how you can use them to achieve your goals, it's time to look at how this can work in practice. We're going to look at the habits and lifestyle of a special group of Buddhist monks – the Shaolin. Even better, Shaolin monks enjoy greater overall wellbeing and a sense of inner peace! It's no wonder that their lifestyle has gradually become an inspiration for many Westerners.

So, who exactly are these exceptional individuals? The Shaolin Monastery in China is one of the most famous Zen Buddhist temples in the world. According to legend, it was founded approximately 1500 years ago when a Buddhist teacher known as Buddhabhadra travelled from India all the way to China. His revolutionary idea was that the core teachings of Buddhism could be passed from a master to student. Until that point, Buddhist monks had usually relied on scriptures and written interpretations. Buddhabhadra's idea impressed the Chinese Emperor, who allocated to him the funds required to build a new temple. The monks were not only trained in spiritual discipline, but also became renowned for their fighting skills. They are taught over 70 special moves including the famous "Iron Head" technique. Those who have perfected this exercise are capable of breaking concrete slabs using just their foreheads. The monks' skills are so impressive that they sometimes tour the world, giving demonstrations to large audiences.

Today, despite numerous attacks and demolitions throughout history, the temple is still home to monks who are famous for their mastery of kung fu. The monks' day starts at 5am and ends at 11pm, with their time split across three main activities – the study of Buddhism, the practicing of kung fu, and essential temple activities such as cleaning and preparing food. Each monk must therefore spend hours each day on grueling physical exercise along with intense mental and spiritual training. Their lifestyle allows for few material possessions and outside interests. Upon joining the temple, each monk is required to shave their head as a sign of their allegiance to the teachings of the Buddha and a symbol of their willingness to give up their attachment to material possessions.

So how do they maintain the high level of self-discipline required to stick to such a strict schedule? According to British-born monk Matthew Ahmet, who trained at the temple for several years, the Shaolin hold a set of attitudes very different to those held in the west. For a start, the monks live with access to only the most basic of facilities, washing their clothes by hand and going without running water. This makes them grateful for even the simplest things in life. This gratitude gives them a positive baseline to work with – when you take time to appreciate the small things, you build psychological momentum. You begin to believe that the world is fundamentally a good place laden with opportunity, which spurs you on to achieve your goals.

Second, the monks know that material possessions and wealth are not the magic key to happiness. They aren't envious of those living "normal" lives because during their training they come to appreciate that real contentment and peace comes from finding a passion or mission. In their case, it's the spiritual and physical progress they make during their time at the temple. This lesson is simple yet powerful – once you find a goal that aligns with your values and ambitions, your passion will carry you a long way. Even when times get hard and it feels as though you still have a long way to go, a sense of purpose can shore up your self-discipline.

Third, they do not believe in pushing themselves to the point of pain or injury. Historically, the monks had to be fit and ready to fight at all times in the event of an attack on their temple. They believed that a monk who was ill or injured as a result of too much physical or mental exertion would be no good in battle. This attitude is still upheld by the modern temple inhabitants. Although the monks spend hours each day in physical training, they also take care to include rest periods in their schedule. They understand that being busy doesn't necessarily equate to being productive. They are taught that sometimes you need to slow down before you burn out. This is where meditation comes in. Ahmet believes that this is the best way to reduce mind chatter, increase your psychological strength, and learn to balance hard work with downtime.

The monks spend hours every day on meditative practices. According to kung fu practitioners, it is important to regulate your emotions and avoid giving into negative impulses. To fight effectively, they believe you must learn how to harness your essential life force. In the Shaolin tradition this is referred to as "chi." Translated from the Chinese, it may mean "air," "energy" or "temper" in English. Monks train for years not only in the high-energy art of kung fu, but they also practice a slow martial art called tai chi. Tai chi is comprised of a collection of physical actions requiring immense concentration and balance. It was developed in order to teach those wishing to learn physical combat how to remain aware and focused in the moment in order to strike quickly and effectively. Shaolin monks attribute their unusual physical toughness, resilience and resistance to injury to this mastery of chi. For example, after a few years of training a typical Shaolin monk will be able to withstand blows to the abdomen and internal organs which would be fatal to anyone else. They use their ability to handle and redirect energy to repel blows and remain uninjured.

Along with granting you the ability to master your chi and quieten your mind, meditation also helps you get in touch with who you really are. This is the most important step in discovering your inner passion and purpose. The Shaolin monks find it easy to get up and go about their day with vigor, because they know exactly what they are going to do and why they are doing it. This inner conviction drives them to physical, mental and spiritual excellence. Although meditation is often thought of as single experience or practice, for Shaolin monks it is a way of life. They aspire to live a life of continual mindfulness and to retain the highest level of concentration at all times.

It should be clear by now that the Shaolin actually have plenty in common with Navy SEALs. Although their day-to-day activities are very different, each monk and SEAL is strongly allied to their particular cause. They all show immense self-discipline and are willing to give up their regular comforts in order to achieve a greater goal. Just as the SEALs don't wake up raring to go each and every morning, the monks probably don't always feel like training for most of the day. However, with such strong ideals and a strict routine to follow, they never need to rely on feeling "motivated." They know how to cultivate a sense of momentum and seeing their skills increase spurs them on still further.

Chapter 14 The Psychology of Self-Discipline

The Special Forces Selection is designed to test the minds and bodies of potential operators. They realized a long time ago that the mind is their most important tool. This is why you too have to master your own psychology to reach your goals and take your life to the next level.

Self-discipline is generally an act of will, so it is important to understand how the human mind works. This is done in order to convert understanding to a greater sense of self-control. Over millions of years, the human being has evolved an even more complex brain. Psychology, as a human endeavor, has shed some light into the mysteries of the mind, finally allowing us to see how things affect or motivate people and how our environment affects how we react to things that occur.

Self-Image

The way people perceive themselves affects how they react to the world. This is shaped by how they have raised and the people that have surrounded them. The environment they grew up in has shaped how they see themselves. There are people with low self-esteem, and this makes them believe that they are unworthy of good things or that they are incapable of achieving perfection.

On the other hand, there are others who have an inflated sense of self-worth, and they believe that they deserve everything without actually having to do much. These people, though they may seem powerful on the outside, are in fact hollow. Cracks in their tough shell will show overwhelming insecurity that they have spent a lifetime hiding. If a man is on the quest to become a true alpha male, he must be able to know the truth about himself and not give in to insecurity or the temptation to take the easy road by simply hiding under a facade.

Locus of Control

A person on the path to self-improvement must find out whether he blames others for the things that happen to him or if he blames himself for what happens to him. If a person blames others all the time for everything that happens, their locus of control is said to be external, which means that they let go of his power to fate or "destiny." This is the weak man's approach, especially if he believes that he is unable to change anything that happens to him. He is weak-minded and weak-willed, and he thinks that whatever happens to him is because of random chance and other people or events. This is a lazy and weak approach to life.

On the other hand, a man whose locus of control is internal tends to see everything as his fault, and if this goes to the extreme, he ends up being too overwhelmed by what is happening to him and even to the world. He might blame himself about something that happened to someone totally unrelated to him. This is unrealistic. We go back to the topic of the self-image: the man must be able to have the right information about himself in order to act upon it.

Classical Conditioning

To challenge the idea that psychology was an armchair pseudoscience, the behaviorist movement, which included the psychologist Ivan Pavlov, brought the scientific method into the field through experimentation. Pavlov was able to show the process of training and conditioning by measuring how much dogs salivated every time a bell was rung to signify food. After the experimenter rings the bell, they put the food out. Soon, even when the experimenter does not bring out food, the mere ringing of the bell makes the dogs react as if they are ready for food. This is called conditioning, and another way to apply this concept is reward and punishment.

People and animals tend to stay from punishment, and they tend to look for rewards. So, rewards will make us keep doing what we were doing in order to get the pleasure of that reward. Punishments work the other way around, so the balance of both reward and punishment will effectively condition a person to a certain kind of action. Because we were born with the capacity to rule ourselves, we can consciously apply this method to ourselves in order to achieve the kind of action we want to learn. Ask yourself how much pain you will get if you don't take action. For example, how much pain will you experience if you don't study for your exam? Maybe you won't graduate. Now think about the short-term pain of studying versus the long-term pain of not graduating. Now think of the reward or pleasure you will get if you do study. You will graduate with a degree and be respected by others. So, in this way, you can trick yourself into doing things that you don't feel like doing.

Psychology of Motivation

When people are asked who will win between a lion and a man in an arena, most people answer the lion because it is more powerful, and it has evolved to be stronger than the man. Unless that man is the mythical Hercules, the lion will no doubt devour him. However, this does not take into consideration the sort of evolution that humanity has gone through in the past millions of years. The human has evolved a more complex brain and the ability to innovate and create weapons. Thus, a fairer fight would be between a lion and a man armed with weapons.

Humans are more complex than animals, and the difference is evident in our desire to become greater than ourselves. This book is already a testament to that. Thus, in motivating a man to become better than himself, it is important that he knows what he is fighting for. He needs a goal, and a way to know whether or not he has achieved it. Not knowing what he is fighting for, even the hardened warrior will fail. A man with a purpose is unstoppable.

Once a person has decided on their goal, they must begin to act. Success is being and doing what you want now, and that can only be achieved if you act immediately and act as if that success is already present now. Soon, even without thinking about it, the goal will have already been reached. It is also important, then, to trust in the process or habit through the continuous application of self-discipline.

Chapter 15 The Triad of Success

We often think of self-esteem and charisma as an immeasurable force or an unknown quality that people have or don't have from birth. It is something we can't look directly at; we can only measure its effects. We can't tell if someone has self-confidence when they are in isolation. Take a confident person, put them in a locked empty room, and you can't measure their true self-esteem. You can only see when you get other people in that room how that person reacts to them.

When we struggle with popularity and leadership, we think of it as this missing essence that we either have or don't have; there is nothing we can do about it because it is hard to measure it within ourselves. I can't determine how self-confidence I am without talking to anyone else, without interacting with other people and seeing how they react. It is hard to figure out how we can improve.

We do know that self-esteem and confidence are core components of charismatic people. People who exude confidence, positive energy and belief in themselves draw people to them. The more you believe in yourself; the more other people believe in you. Look at leaders throughout history – even misguided leaders. They had a powerful force because they believed in themselves so much that even when they were wrong, people followed them. That is the power of their self-esteem and self-belief.

Before you can build up confidence in your ability to do things, you have to build up your belief in yourself, your self-esteem, and how much you like yourself. It is hard to push yourself for greatness when you don't like yourself, when you don't believe in yourself, and when you don't think that you are good enough.

Things to Think About

1. Think about the most confident people you know; it can be people in your life or people on television. You can look at great leaders throughout history. I used to know someone in college who loved to listen to great speeches from history. He thought if that he listened to enough speeches by leaders, it would eventually turn him in a leader. It did not work.

Take a look at some of the most confident people in your life and from history and then assess their confidence. Do you notice something in common? When you look at specific examples, you will start to see how there is a strong correlation between confidence and charisma in people. Not every competent person becomes charismatic, but every charismatic person certainly has a great deal of confidence that they project in the world.

Are you beginning to see the link between confidence and charisma? If you think I am dead wrong, that is okay; write that down in your Love Yourself Journal. It is okay to disagree with me and to begin to push yourself and start thinking about these ideas. This is all about helping your thought process evolve.

2. Take some time to reflect on the reasons for the link between confidence and charisma. Why do you think confidence helps us seem more charismatic to other people? When you think of someone you know in your actual life **that** is charismatic, do you think their confidence is what pulled you into their orbit?

3. Now that you have been with me on this journey for a little bit, do you feel more comfortable and excited about this process? Do you have some specific action steps that you are planning to take to move you further along this process to become more didtic? Perhaps you have already taken some of the steps.

4. Think back to a time when you met someone who had very low **self-confidence** or maybe a moment where someone revealed a deep lack of self-confidence. Did you notice a corresponding lack of self-esteem? At the time, were you repulsed or repelled by the force of their low self-confidence? Now that you have a better understanding, do you understand why we pull away from people with low self-confidence? Do you think differently about the situation now than you did at the time?

Reflecting on the Past Exercise

We are now going to go through eight scenarios, and I want you to reflect on each of them. Think of a time when you experienced each scenario and write your answers in your Love Yourself Journal.

1. Think of a time when your lack of confidence blocked you from convincing other people to take action. Maybe you were just trying to convince your friend to see a certain movie with you but you weren't sure that the movie would be good, or you weren't sure that you were making the right choice, and rather than taking people to a move they might not like, you let someone else decide and saw a movie that you didn't like. Whatever your example is, write it down in your Love Yourself Journal.

2. Think of a time when your lack of confidence kept you from asserting yourself when you should have spoken up or taken action. Maybe you have one of those stories from high school which we all have, when people were picking on someone, and you wished you had said something to stop them.

3. Think of a time when your lack of self-confidence stopped you from pursuing a goal. Did you want to pursue athletics into college? Did you want to pursue an artistic career and didn't think you were good

enough? Maybe you did not believe that you had what it takes to go to the next level.

4. Did your lack of confidence interfere with your education? I had a friend who was significantly smarter than me. He was a self-taught autodidact, played five instruments, and was offered a full scholarship to college but didn't go; he thought he was too dumb. He was convinced that he wasn't good enough and he froze his education. Do you have an experience like this in your own life?

5. How about a time when your lack of confidence interfered with your career? Maybe you didn't apply for a job you could have gotten, or you didn't ask your boss for the promotion or say, "You don't need to hire someone else; I can do it."

6. Can you think of a time you felt frustrated? A time where your self-esteem was trapped inside you and you could not express yourself the way you wanted to. You couldn't put together the right words or emotions – you felt trapped in your head, and you could not communicate with the world in the way you wanted to.

7. Do you ever feel trapped in a cycle, going from low self-confidence to low self-esteem and back and forth again? People don't listen to what you have to say. They say negative things about you, and they say that you are not a good leader. They might say you don't

know how to handle yourself, so you feel bad and stop believing yourself.

Maybe have not always been in the cycle, but perhaps there has been a time in your life when you felt trapped in it. Analyze how you felt in that moment and how you feel looking back at that moment.

Confidence and Self-Esteem Experiment Exercise

There is another self-esteem and confidence technique that I have not shared with you yet. This technique is very powerful; I have implemented it in the past, and it was for transformative for me. It works very well in complement with the territory-based confidence technique. Maybe you have heard this term before; it is called "fakes it until you make it." Understanding how this process works is the key to its success.

In your Journal, create version 2.0 of yourself. If you have read one of my other books where you have done the process before, it may be time for you to do a 3.0 version. Describe a version of yourself that has super high levels of competence and self-esteem. Describe the person that you wish you were. Imagine you are six months in the future and describe yourself in great detail. Create a three-dimensional character in your mind and then write every detail down in your Love Yourself Journal. This version 2.0 is the ultimate in self-esteem and confidence – the person you wish you were.

Once you've created this character and have a firm feeling of what confidence looks like when applied to you, you have to spend the next week pretending to be this person. You are going to be an actor for seven days, pretending to be your 2.0 or 3.0. You are playing a role, so you constantly have to ask yourself, "What would 2.0 say or do?"

Spend a week seeing how this character acts. You may go through a phase where you go too far in the other direction, and I've done this myself. I emulated a specific super-confident version of myself that was too far and became a jerk, so I calibrated down the following week. That's okay. It's better to push too far and then bring it back a little bit rather than spend the rest of your life wondering if you added enough confidence.

Pretend to be this person for a week. Every time someone asks you a question, you say what your 2.0 would say. At the end of each day, when you get home, open your Love Yourself Journal and respond to the following questions:

1. Did people treat you differently, as if you were more confident? How did it feel acting like a different person throughout the day?

2. How much do you feel that your change in self-confidence affected your self-esteem? Did pretending to be more confident actually make you a person with a high self-esteem level? Can false confidence create self-esteem?

3. Now that you have gone through this exercise pretending to be more confident, do you actually feel more confident? Do you feel like you made actual permanent changes to your confidence and self-esteem levels?

4. Do you feel that this exercise has improved your self-esteem?

5. Will you continue this exercise for the long term? Do you feel this exercise can become a permanent part of your life?

If you spend enough time pretending to be a better version of yourself, you will become that person. This is a very powerful technique. It starts at the opposite end of the spectrum. This technique starts with your interactions with other people; it starts with the outermost shell of your personality.

When combined with our territory-based confidence technique, which starts at your core, the process is twice as fast. These techniques work very well in tandem. They are unbelievably powerful.

6. Are you going to stick with this technique and continue to use it? Do you like seeing how the benefits work? Would you like to be this person all the time without doing it on purpose?

7. If someone walked up to right now and said, "You read that amazing book. How can I become more self-

confident?" What would you tell them to do? What action steps would you give to someone else who wants to become more confident?

Chapter 16 Making Things Pleasurable and Fun!

One of the cool things that may continue to motivate you towards becoming more disciplined is learning that people who are able to master these skills turn out to be happier in general! Self-discipline isn't about simply avoiding things that feel temporarily good, but also about being able to avoid things that eventually make you feel worse. Disciplined people can think farther ahead and see that acting on a whim causes a cascade of negative outcomes and that these negative outcomes will have a sense of lack of control and less happiness.

Disciplined people can see two conflicting situations: desire to complete a task that is hard vs desire to quit and do fun things. Research has found a strong correlation between those that complete tasks and can stay dedicated to those tasks and higher satisfaction in life. This seems quite intuitive as those people also tend to accomplish things that improve their life. Research also shows that the ability to stick to completing tasks means less influence by negative emotions at all and more time feeling positive or calm.

These people weren't better able to resist an impulse or temptation, but rather were better at designing a life that didn't introduce as many of those temptations in the first place. They were better at crafting a life situation that didn't include those cravings, distractions or sabotaging behaviors. Instead of simply "being stronger" than others, those who are disciplined just avoid finding themselves in situations that create conflict with their stated goals.

But what if you really do thrive off fun? Let's work that into your goals as well! Nobody said that discipline had to be sacrifice and pain with no reward. We simply need to remove rewards that turn into distractions for yourself.

Start by making a list of rewards you enjoy. After you list the things that feel rewarding, ask yourself:

- Do these ever take me away from my goals, like a piece of candy when I'm trying to lose weight?

- Do I struggle to moderate this if I engage in it?

If you answer yes to either of those two situations, they will be short term rewards that turn into long term distractions. If they don't distract, then feel free to use them! An example is using the Pomodoro technique we talked about earlier. At the end of each dedicated time, you can have a treat, if you aren't prone to overeating. Or if you still want that reward, portion out an exact amount and put the rest far away from where you are working. Or if social media is your reward, then set a new timer for your reward time and set a commitment to stop when the timer is up. If you find that you try a reward and you can't stop or stay distracted, it's time to make that your FINAL ending reward once you finish the task. This way your work is already done, and since it's a one-time reward and not something you keep doing intermittently until the task is done, you may find it easier to moderate.

You can also find that the very things that motivate you are also fun! Motivation is typically a positive emotion, that comes with a surge of excitement. Do you need to watch motivational video's every day? Follow people on social media who inspire you? Listen to songs as you work that help you feel energized to work or complete a workout? The nice thing about motivating yourself is that you don't find it to be an energy drain! The very things that motivate you may jump start you each day to complete your tasks!

Never forget as well that the product of your work will be reward, but that can also be true daily. Your ability to go out and have fun is even more of a reward when done after completing tasks that make you feel accomplished! If you can see dedication and discipline as motivating and invigorating instead of draining and a pain, you can find it far more engaging and easier to do! It all goes back to

Conclusion

Self-discipline is something that will take time for you to master. There are no shortcuts and no definite tips that will help you to achieve your goals overnight. However, if you remain dedicated to the process and make small strides each day, you will find that you are going to be more likely to be able to reach the goals that you set for yourself.

You can even start working on your goals at home and then watch them spill over into your professional life. This can begin by taking steps to do more around the home or even exercising at night while you are watching television.

With the tips that are listed in this book, the chances of you being successful are going to increase dramatically. It will be important that you routinely review these tips from time to time and begin to explore the tips that help you the most. Many of the tips can work in a number of areas of your life and you can combine tips to maximize their effectiveness. If you do find something isn't a match for you, consider some of the others in the book instead. That way, you maximize the benefit your benefit from this collection.